The Female Electrocardiogram

Pentti M. Rautaharju

The Female Electrocardiogram

Special Repolarization Features, Gender Differences, and the Risk of Adverse Cardiac Events

Springer

Pentti M. Rautaharju
Division of Public Health Sciences
Wake Forest School of Medicine
Winston-Salem, NC
USA

ISBN 978-3-319-15292-9 ISBN 978-3-319-15293-6 (eBook)
DOI 10.1007/978-3-319-15293-6

Library of Congress Control Number: 2015934580

Springer Cham Heidelberg New York Dordrecht London

Printed on acid-free paper

Springer International Publishing AG Switzerland is part of Springer Science+Business Media (www.springer.com)

Dedicated to my wife Dr. Farida Rautaharju, who collaborated with me for over a quarter of a century in operating EPICARE, a core ECG center for epidemiological studies and clinical trials.

Preface

Happy Hearts and Broken Hearts

In many industrialized countries including the USA, cardiovascular disease (CVD) continues to be the leading cause of death. Early epidemiological and clinical studies on coronary heart disease (CHD) focused almost exclusively on men. CHD was considered to be a male disease, and women's health issues had a low priority. Political pressure gradually changed the situation, and as a result, major research programs addressing women's health issues were introduced, such as the large-scale Women's Health Initiative (WHI) study in 1991. Since then, women have been increasingly included in CHD intervention efforts, but substantial gender differences still remain in CVD prevalence and mortality. The number of heart attacks or fatal CHD annually in women equals that in men but with a shift in time by 10 years. Differences in population demographics account for the fact that in terms of absolute numbers, more women than men are living with and dying from CHD, and more women than men are discharged from hospitals with diagnosis of heart failure and stroke.

Electrocardiography plays an important role in prevention of CHD and in prevention of adverse cardiac events associated with CHD. New ECG predictors for CHD morbidity and mortality have recently emerged. The goal of this monograph is to examine closer these new promising predictors. The primary objective is to evaluate gender differences in special ECG features and in ECG predictors for the risk of adverse cardiac events and to explore mechanisms for gender differences in risk predictors.

The noble mission of medicine is to alleviate pain and preferably to prevent the disease causing the suffering. Among the challenging missions of cardiovascular medicine is to prevent CHD and CVD. Improved knowledge of gender differences and special features in female electrocardiogram will help in this task. Substantial progress has been made in improving therapeutic actions to treat patients in conditions such as acute coronary syndrome (ACS) and heart attack caused by CHD. CHD preventive efforts are also gradually, albeit slowly, bringing tangible results. Genetic, neurohormonal, and environmental factors involved in CHD, CVD, and SCD are complex, as is life itself. Well-balanced harmony of these factors makes a happy heart, and at the other extreme, death from a broken heart has been documented to occur in prolonged excessive sympathetic overdrive in uncontrolled grief.

Weston, FL, USA Pentti M. Rautaharju

Acknowledgement

I wish to acknowledge the collaboration of the present and former staff members and directors of the EPICARE Center, particularly Dr. Zhu-ming Zhang, Dr. Ronald J. Prineas, and Dr. Elsayed Soliman. The EPICARE Center, initially at Dalhousie University and the University of Alberta, Canada, and since 1994 at Wake Forest University School of Medicine, NC, has been in charge of ECG analysis for all major national health surveys of the National Center for Health Statistics and United States Centers for Disease Control and Prevention and for many collaborative clinical trials sponsored by NIH, such as the Multiple Risk Factor Intervention Trial (MRFIT), the Women's Health Initiative (WHI), Cardiovascular Health Study (CHS), and the Arteriosclerosis Risk in Communities (ARIC) study.

I also wish to express my appreciation and gratitude to Dr. Henry Blackburn, my friend and collaborator during the formative and formidable years of my graduate studies at the University of Minnesota in the early 1960s, when the foundations of epidemiological electrocardiography were laid. It is worth noting that according to the citation index, the Minnesota code paper (Blackburn H et al. *Circulation*. 1960;21:1160–75) was still in 2012 among the four most frequently cited articles in electrocardiographic literature.

Contents

Chapter 1
Special Features of the Female Electrocardiogram

Synopsis This chapter presents brief introductory notes about some special features of the female electrocardiogram (ECG). ECGs are generally displayed as one-dimensional functions of time with different ECG leads grouped in various conventional sequences to provide some two-dimensional (2-D) information such as chest leads V1 through V6. The mean horizontal plane (XZ) QRS and T vector loops of normal adult women show that the spatial direction of the initial repolarization sequence in horizontal plane is predominantly reverse and terminal repolarization concordant with depolarization sequence. Frontal plane QRS and T vector loops both are narrow and directed to the left indicating that spatial direction of repolarization sequence in frontal plane is predominantly reverse with respect to depolarization sequence.

Two-dimensional display of vector loops in principal planes is reasonably effective for illustrating ECG data of an individual person or mean ECG data of a group of individuals. However, these display formats reveal no information about the scatter or clustering of directional information at various time points of excitation or repolarization sequence. Directional distributions of vectorial data require in essence three-dimensional displays. Novel three-dimensional display procedures are introduced in this chapter for this purpose. Of particular importance is information obtained about three-dimensional distribution at time points of peak QRS peak and T peak vectors. While the spatial distribution of T peak vector is relatively tightly clustered at time point T peak and remain tightly clustered throughout repolarization, spatial directions of QRS vectors vary widely in the course of depolarization. The latter finding corresponds to QRS vectors rotating over 180° through the depolarization sequence.

Among the most characteristic features in female ECG with distinctive gender differences are ST segment patterns in anterior chest leads particularly in V2. The ST segment amplitude increases slowly from the J-point (end of QRS) until the onset of the T wave and then increases more rapidly until T wave peak. The slowly ascending ST segment with a relatively tall positive T wave in V2 represents a characteristic female ('U'-shaped) waveform with a positive convexity.

P.M. Rautaharju, *The Female Electrocardiogram: Special Repolarization Features, Gender Differences, and the Risk of Adverse Cardiac Events*,
DOI 10.1007/978-3-319-15293-6_1

Abbreviations and Acronyms

AL	Anterior-left
AR	Anterior-right
AS	Anterior-superior
ILA	Inferior-left-anterior
IP	Inferior-posterior
IRA	Inferior-right-anterior
L	Left
PL	Posterior-left
PR	Posterior-right
R	Right
Rp	R wave peak
RT	Repolarization time
RTgrad	RT gradient
SLP	Superior-left-posterior
SRP	Superior-right-posterior
Tp	T wave peak

1.1 Electrocardiographic and Vectorcardiographic Patterns of Adult Women

The main characteristics of the electrocardiogram of normal adult women are presented in this chapter, with a special focus on those ECG features where the sex differences are most pronounced. Sex differences will be covered in detail in Chap. 3.

The chest lead ECGs V1-V6 in Fig. 1.1 of a normal 57 year old woman show the normal gradual transition of QRS from rS patterns (small initial R and large S waves) in V1 and V2 to qR pattern (small Q and tall R waves) in left lateral lead V6. T wave amplitude in V1 can normally be negative, biphasic (negative/positive) or flat as in this ECG. TV2 is generally positive but it can occasionally be slightly negative. In other chest leads T wave amplitudes are normally positive.

P waves in leads II, V1 and aVR are shown on an enlarged scale in Fig. 1.2. The P waves are seen merging with some overlap into atrial repolarization (so called Ta wave). The PR interval in this ECG was measured as 178 ms. The onset of the QRS complex cuts the Ta wave short. P wave in V1 is biphasic with the initial positive deflection corresponding to the right atrial depolarization and the terminal negative deflection corresponding to the left atrial depolarization in left-posterior direction. Increased terminal PV1 amplitude and duration are used in criteria for left atrial overload. The spatial sequence of atrial repolarization is closely concordant with the spatial direction of atrial depolarization sequence. Because cardiac membrane current flow during repolarization is reverse with respect to the depolarization current flow, Ta waves are of opposite polarity compared to the P waves.

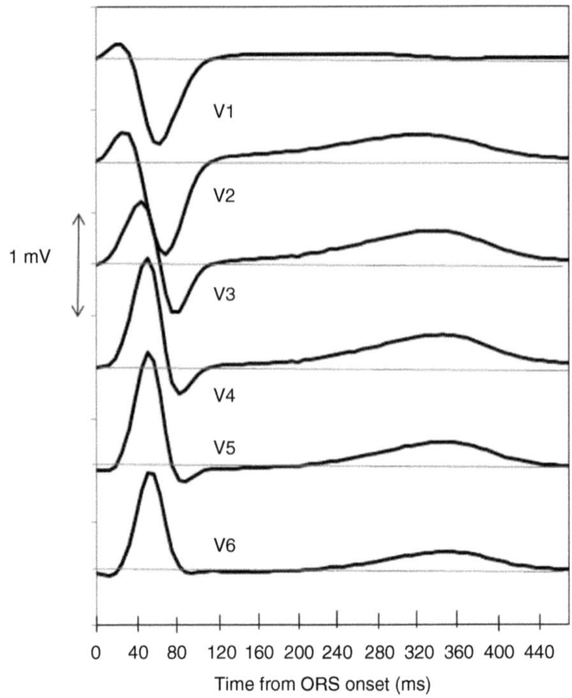

Fig. 1.1 ECG Chest leads V1–V3 and V4–V6 of a normal 57 years old woman

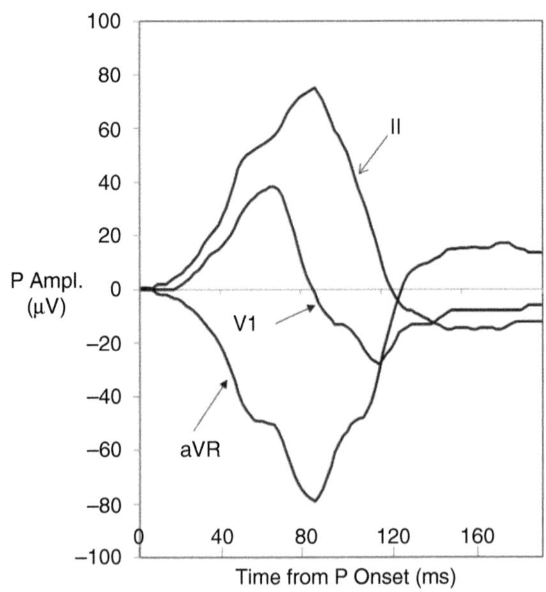

Fig. 1.2 P waves in leads II, V1 and aVR of the ECG in Fig. 1.1 shown on an enlarged scale. Initial portion of atrial repolarization with opposite polarity to that of the P waves is seen until the end of the PR interval (measured as 178 ms) before the onset of QRS

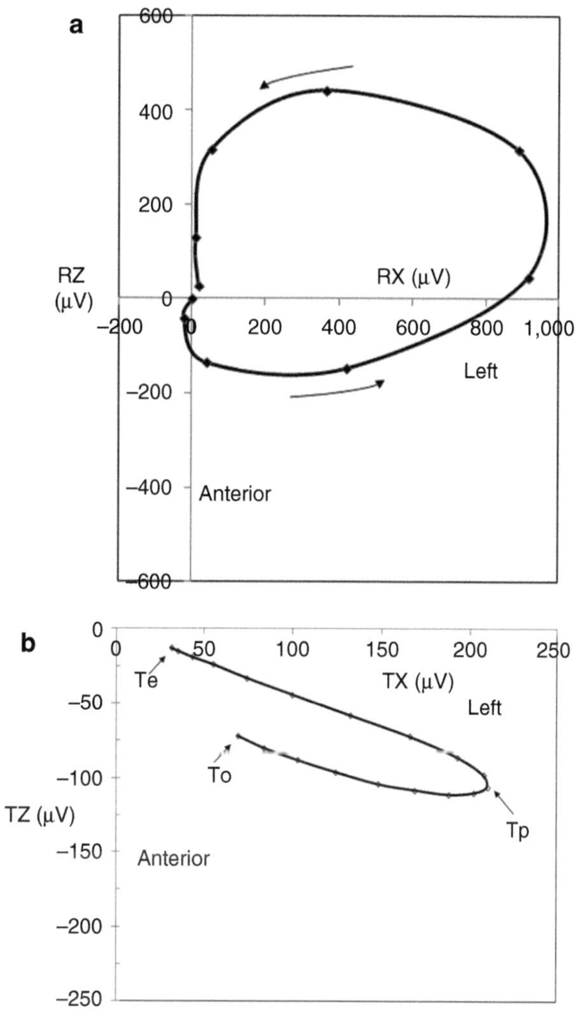

Fig. 1.3 The mean horizontal (XZ) plane QRS vector loop (**a**) and T vector loop (**b**) of normal adult women. The spatial direction of initial repolarization sequence in horizontal plane is predominantly reverse and terminal repolarization concordant with depolarization sequence

Figure 1.3 shows the mean horizontal plane (XZ) QRS vector loop (a) and T vector loop (b) of normal adult women. During initial repolarization T amplitudes are concordant (same polarity) with QRS amplitudes and during terminal half discordant which indicates that the spatial direction of initial repolarization sequence in horizontal plane is predominantly reverse and terminal repolarization concordant with depolarization sequence.

Figure 1.4 shows the mean frontal plane (XZ) QRS vector loop (a) and T vector loop (b). The QRS and T vector loops both are narrow and directed to the left indicating that spatial direction of repolarization sequence in frontal plane is predominantly reverse with respect to depolarization sequence.

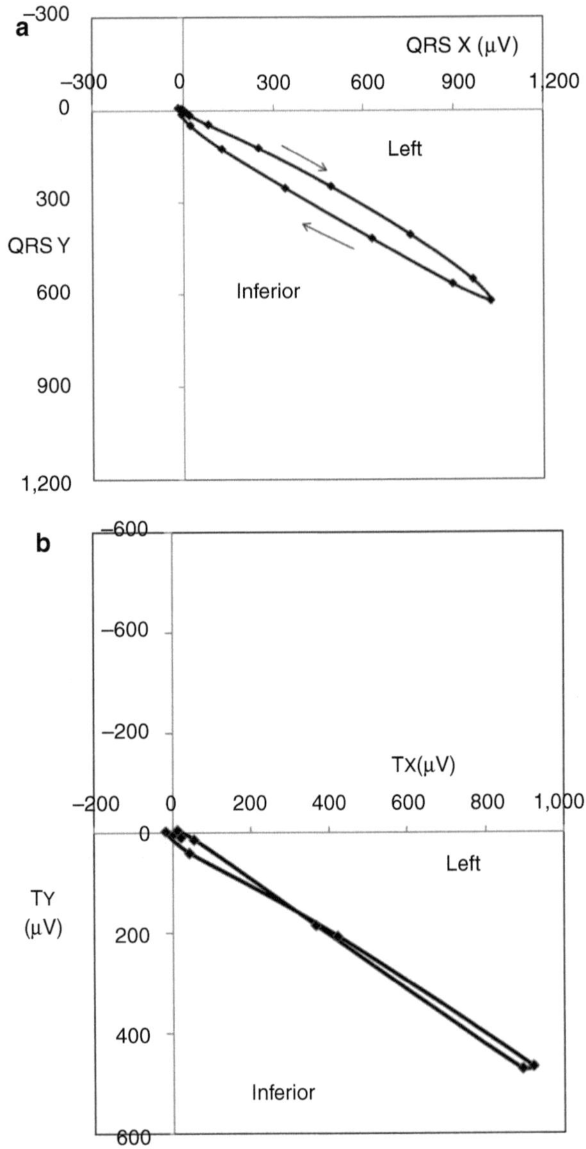

Fig. 1.4 The mean frontal (XZ) plane QRS vector loop (**a**) and T vector loop (**b**). The QRS and T vector loops both are narrow and directed to the left indicating that spatial direction of repolarization sequence in frontal plane is predominantly reverse with respect to depolarization sequence

1.2 Spatial Directions of Normal Excitation and Repolarization Sequences in Women

Although vector loops such as the QRS loops and T vector loops are fairly effective in displaying 2-D data of an individual or the mean data, they reveal no information about the scatter or clustering of directional information at various time points of excitation or repolarization sequence. Directional distributions of vectorial data

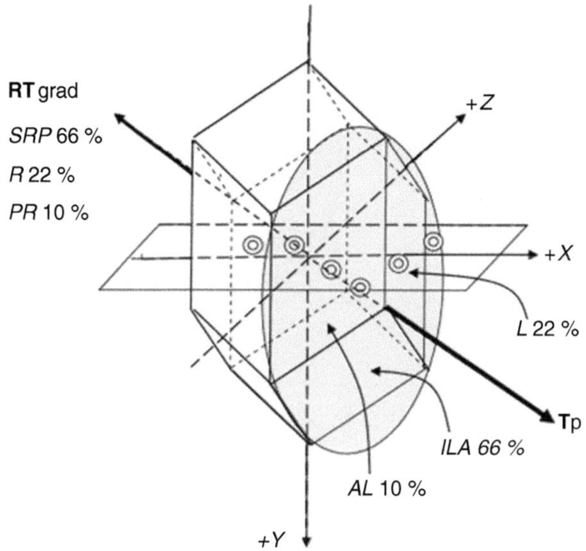

Fig. 1.5 Spatial directions of T peak (Tp) vectors in normal women shown in a spatial rhombic duododecahedron reference frame. The orientation of 96 % of the vectors is within 3 out of 12 rhombic spatial reference zones (enclosed within the *circle shaded light green*). The labels for the directions are listed in order of the prevalence as Inferior-Left-Anterior (ILA), Left (L) or Anterior-Left (AL) direction. Repolarization time gradient (RTgrad) vectors indicate spatial orientation of the repolarization sequence which are diametrically opposite to the direction of the Tp vectors. Double rings show the approximate spatial directions of the lead vectors of the chest leads V1 V6, with Wilson's central terminal at the intersection of X, Y and Z axis (From Rautaharju et al. [1])

require in essence three-dimensional displays such as the shown for the distributions of Tpeak (Tp) vectors in normal women in Fig. 1.5. The figure shows 12 rhombic faces distributed equally in 12 spatial directions. It is noted that in 96 % Tp directions are clustered within 3 of the 12 spatial directions, rhombic faces labeled ILA, AL and L referring to inferior-left-anterior, anterior-left and left in order of directional dominance, respectively. While the direction of excitation sequence at time point of QRS peak (Rp) vector is the same as the direction of the spatial excitation sequence, the spatial direction of repolarization sequence is diametrically opposite to Tp vector direction because the membrane current flow in cardiac myocytes during repolarization is reverse with respect to the direction of current flow during depolarization. Spatial direction of repolarization is represented by the temporal repolarization time (RT) gradient vector labeled RTgrad. Thus, RTgrad directions are opposite to Tp vectors, in directions SRP, PR and R referring to superior-right-posterior, posterior-right and right, respectively. Spatial direction of repolarization remains consistently throughout repolarization within the three reference directions of RTgrad vector.

While a 3-D display such as in Fig. 1.5 is informative, it is impractical for more widely clustered distributions and it also does not show distributions in posterior

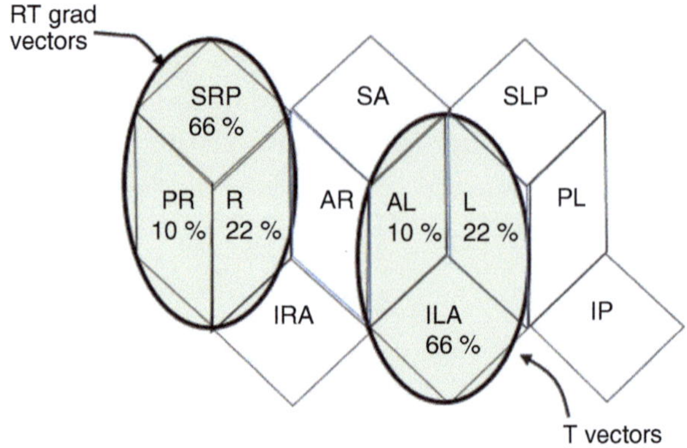

Fig. 1.6 Clusters of the distributions of Tp and the corresponding RTgrad vectors in normal adult women shown the 3-D rhombic lattice in Fig. 1.5 opened up in midposterior line and projecting the rhombic faces as a 2-D display in the frontal plane

orientation without 3-D rotation of the rhombic lattice. A practical solution for displaying 3-D vector distributions is to open up the 3-D rhombic lattice in midposterior line and project the rhombic faces as a 2-D display of undistorted rhombic faces in frontal plane. Figure 1.6 shows the distributions of Tp and the corresponding RTgrad distributions in normal adult women.

While the spatial directions of Tp and RTgrad are relatively tightly clustered at time point Tp and remain tightly clustered in these same three directions throughout repolarization, spatial directions of QRS vectors vary widely in the course of depolarization as can be deduced already from the horizontal plane QRS vector loop in Fig. 1.2 with mean QRS vectors rotating over 180°. A 2-D display of QRS vector distributions in normal women is shown in Fig. 1.7 for three different Deciles of depolarization. The initial Decile is labeled one tenth, the midpoint five tenth and the terminal nine tenth. The large oval in center-left of the figure shows the distribution of excitation sequence directions at the initial Decile containing 86 % of QRS vectors. The dominant directions are AR (45 %) and AL (20 %), with SA in 13 % and IRA in 8 %. The remaining 14 % were scattered outside the large oval. The relatively large directional variation of the initial QRS vectors reflects the variations in the distributions of the main fascicles of the left bundle branch and the Purkinje network at the septal left ventricular surface. The smaller ellipse in middle-left of the figure shows the anterior-leftwards shift of the QRS vectors from the initial to the mid Decile of QRS. The rightmost oval in the figure shows the major cluster of the terminal QRS vector distributions, with 62 % directed to PL (45 %) or IP (17 %). The second smaller cluster of the terminal QRS vector directions is oriented to PR (21 %) or SRP (10 %).

Considering the stationarity in the spatial orientation of the repolarization sequence in Fig. 1.6, the large variations in the spatial QRS|T angle described in later chapters are largely due to varying orientation of the normal depolarization sequence.

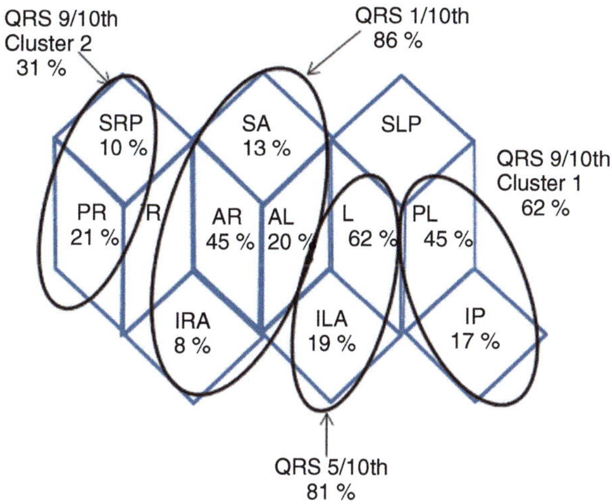

Fig. 1.7 Ovals showing the main clusters of the spatial distributions of the QRS vectors at QRS duration Deciles labeled one tenth, five tenth, nine tenth of QRS. QRS vector orientation during Decile 1 is scattered, mainly to anterior right (45 % and anterior left (20 %), superior-anterior in 13 % and inferior-right-anterior in 8 %, apparently depending on the distribution of the Purkinje network at left ventricular septal surface. The QRS vector orientation clustering is tight at half-way of depolarization (Decile 5). Decile 9 forms two main clusters, with the main cluster 1 oriented to posterior-left or inferior-posterior and the smaller cluster 2 to posterior-right or superior-right-posterior. Considering that T vector orientation and repolarization sequence remains stationary in normal repolarization, the spatial QRS/angle is largely dependent of normal variations of the QRS vector orientation during depolarization

1.3 ST-T Waveform Patterns in Normal Adult Women

The graph in Fig. 1.8 shows the ST-T waveform pattern in lead V5 of a normal adult woman. The ST segment amplitude increases slowly from the J-point (end of QRS) until the onset of the T wave (To) and then increases more rapidly until T wave peak (Tp). Definitions for the convexity (C) of the J-Tp segment are often confusing. In the repolarization model convexity is defined so that it is independent of the polarity of the lead [1]. Convexity is measured as the largest distance of the J-Tp curve from the gradient line drawn from the J-point to Tp. With this definition the convexity of a 'U-shaped' J-Tp segment is positive (ST curve below the gradient line) and a 'dome-shaped' J-Tp negative (ST curve above gradient line). Slowly ascending ST segment with a tall positive T wave has a high positive convexity as in this figure. A similar pattern in commonly observed in leads V3 to V5 of normal women. This graph is presented here because the STT patterns particularly in lead V2 are among the main features with prominent sex differences covered in detail in Chap. 2.

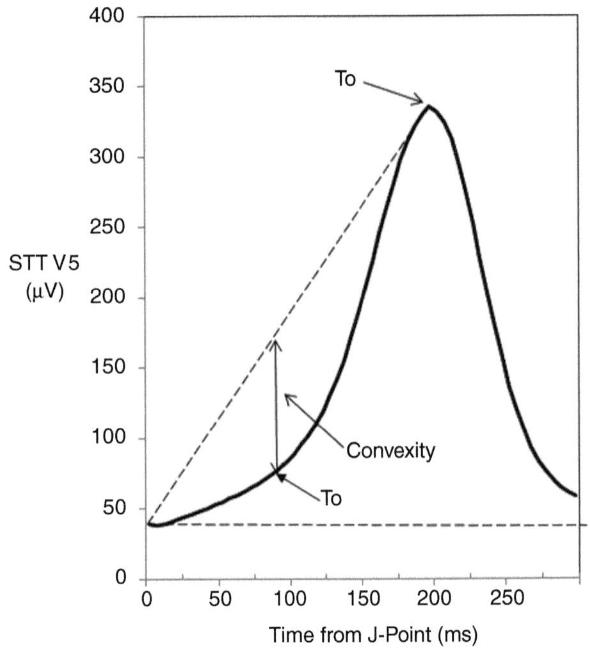

Fig. 1.8 ST-T waveform pattern in lead V5 of a normal adult woman. The ST segment amplitude increases slowly from the J-point (end of QRS) until the onset of the T wave (To) and then increases more rapidly until T wave peak (Tp). Convexity (C) is measured as positive or negative value of the largest distance of the J-Tp curve from the line drawn from the J-point to Tp. A 'U-shaped' J-Tp curve is positive and a 'dome-shaped' J-Tp is negative

Reference

1. Rautaharju PM, et al. Electrocardiographic estimates of regional action potential durations and repolarization time subintervals reveal ischemia-induced abnormalities in acute coronary syndrome not evident from global QT. J Electrocardiol. 2011;44:718–24.

Chapter 2
Gender Differences Emerging During Adolescence in Heart Rate, QRS Duration, QT Interval and ST Elevation

Synopsis QRS duration, heart rate, ST elevation and QT interval are the female ECG features with profound and consistent differences from those in male ECG. Sex differences are small in young children until adolescence but are evolving rapidly during adolescence reflecting profound dynamic hemodynamic, anatomic structural and electrophysiological changes and remodeling. QRS duration in adolescent girls is 6 ms shorter and heart rate 5 bpm faster than in adolescent boys and the difference persists through adulthood. A substantial gender difference in ST amplitudes particularly in anterior chest lead V2 emerges during adolescence due to ST amplitude increase in boys. The gender difference remains significant in all age groups of adults although ST amplitudes gradually decrease in men with age. ST elevation levels in African-Americans are higher than those in white men and women, and ST elevation in African-American men is particularly pronounced. Rate-adjusted QT shortens in adolescent boys with only minor change in girls and QT remains shorter in men than in women through adulthood. Neurohormonal factors primarily testosterone appear as likely common mechanisms of gender differences in the evolution of ST elevation and QT. The mechanism for the higher ST amplitudes in African-American than in white women and men remains open.

Abbreviations and Acronyms

ARIC	Arteriosclerosis research in communities
CVD	Cardiovascular disease
LV	Left ventricular
RT	Repolarization time
RTendo	Endocardial repolarization time
RTepi	Epicardial repolarization time

P.M. Rautaharju, *The Female Electrocardiogram: Special Repolarization Features, Gender Differences, and the Risk of Adverse Cardiac Events*,
DOI 10.1007/978-3-319-15293-6_2

2.1 Evolution with Age of Heart Rate, QRS Duration and QT Interval

This chapter covers gender differences in age- evolution of QT and other main ECG features during adolescence. The main focus of this chapter will be on sex differences in ST elevation and depression. QT evolution with age and the mechanisms for sex differences in QT will be covered in detail in Chap. 9 of this Monograph.

The evolution and the appearance of sex differences in QRS duration and heart rate was documented in a Canadian pediatric material [1] and confirmed in a larger normal study population by Mason et al. [2] covering a wide age range of children and adults (Table 2.1). QRS duration in age groups 15–19 and 20–29 years was 6 ms shorter and heart rate was 5 bpm faster in women than in men. Sex differences in QRS duration are further highlighted in Fig. 2.1.

The rate-adjusted QT is commonly thought to be due to QT prolongation in women. A Canadian investigation on the age-evolution of QT reported in 1992 that gender difference in rate-adjusted QT arises from QT shortening in adolescent males rather than QT prolongation in females [3] (Fig. 2.2). The findings of the Canadian study were confirmed by a more recent study in a large group of women and men covering a wide age range [4]. The observed shorter QT in men than in women is unexpected because QRS duration is longer in men than in women reflecting higher left ventricular mass. More recent studies have demonstrated that the shorter rate-adjusted QT in men than in women is associated with an earlier start and earlier end of left ventricular (LV) epicardial repolarization [5, 6]. Data from Rautaharju et al. [7] in Table 3.2 in Chap. 3 will show that LV epicardial repolarization time (RTepi) is shorter in men than in women. QRS duration does not contribute to LV lateral wall RTepi or endocardial RT (RTendo) because of the reverse sequence of repolarization. However, QRS duration still contributes to QT prolongation during the terminal repolarization which is predominantly concordant with respect to depolarization sequence.

Table 2.1 Heart rate and QRS duration in normal men and women by age

	Sample size		Heart rate (bpm)		QRS duration (ms)	
	Women	Men	Women	Men	Women	Men
5–9	335	524	86±13.5	82±12.3	77±9.5	80±9.8
10–14	259	443	76±11.9	75±12.1^NS†^	83±9.5	84±10^NS^
15–19	310	333	70±12.0	65±11.0	89±8.7	95±8.8
20–29	2,469	2,528	69±11.3	64±11.7	89±9.4	95±9.3
30–39	3,954	3,411	70±11.0	67±11.7	89±9.5	94±9.4
40–49	7,633	5,362	70±11.0	68±11.6	88±9.3	94±9.4
50–59	6,340	5,344	69±11.2	69±12.0^NS^	88±9.6	94±9.3
60–69	5,067	4,466	68±11.4	68±12.3^NS^	88±9.4	94±9.6
70–79	3,745	2,901	67±10.9	65±11.6	87±9.6	93±9.7
80–89	1,291	864	67±10.8	64±11.0	88±10.0	93±9.6

Modified from Rautaharju et al. [4]

NS signifies P<0.05 for t-test for the difference between the mean values of women and men; other differences were significant (P<0.001 for all)

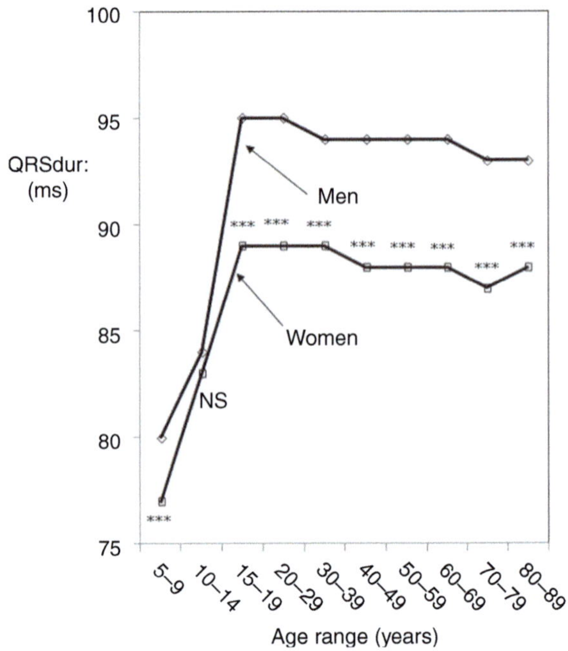

Fig. 2.1 Evolution of QRS duration with age showing the appearance of gender differences during adolescence and prevailing through adulthood although gradually diminishing in magnitude with age (From Rautaharju et al. [4] with permission)

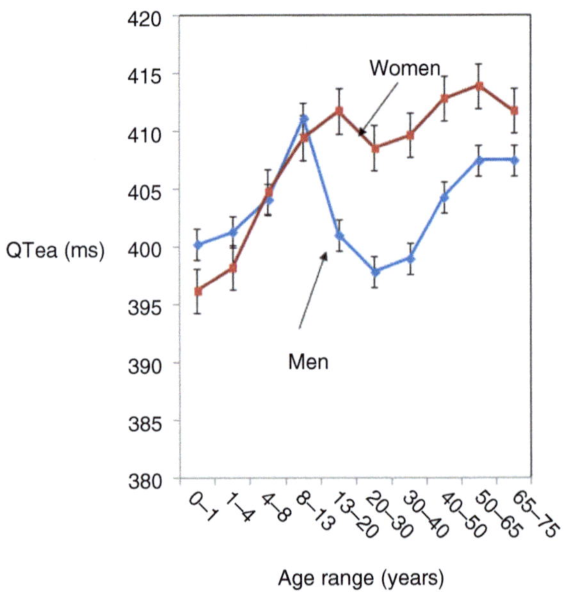

Fig. 2.2 Evolution of the rate-adjusted QTend interval with age showing the appearance of gender differences during adolescence persisting during adulthood although gradually diminishing in magnitude (From Rautaharju et al. [3])

A more detailed evaluation of sex differences in QT evolution in Chap. 9 shows that neurohormonal factors primarily testosterone appear as likely common mechanisms of gender differences in the evolution of ST elevation and QT.

2.2 Gender Differences in the Evolution with Age of ST J-Point Amplitude

Ezaki et al. documented gender differences in the age-evolution of ST amplitudes in a study population of 640 subjects from 5 to 89 years in age [8]. These investigators observed a profound increase in STJ-point amplitude in men in age group 15–19 years with no increase in women in this age group or older. The sex difference decreased after age 30 years because ST amplitudes in men decreased gradually in men but ST segment amplitudes in men remained significantly higher in men than in women in all age groups of adults.

Rijnbeek et al. documented normal values derived from a large group (N = 13,354) of Dutch clinically normal men and women ranging in age from 19 to 90 years [9]. Figure 2.3 adapted from Supplementary Table 8 of that report shows the median values of the ST J-point amplitudes by age in women and men. The graphs show that J-point amplitude in adolescent males is distinctly higher than in females, confirming the observation of Ezaki et al. As in Ezaki's report, the gender difference in J-point amplitude gradually levels off in older age groups.

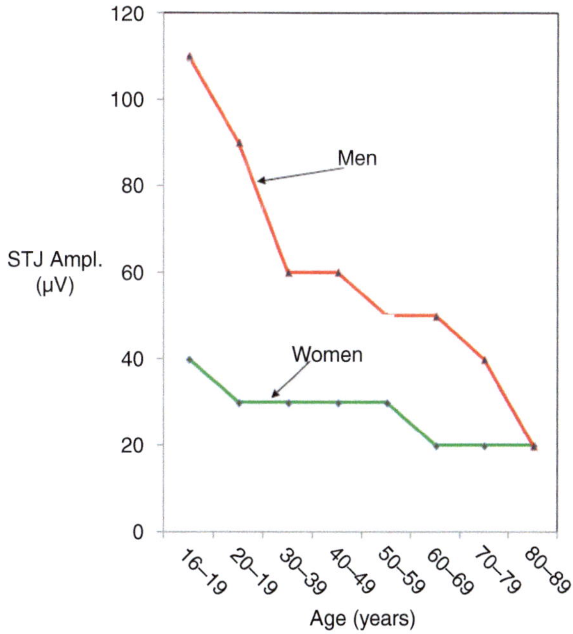

Fig. 2.3 Age-evolution of the median values of ST J-point amplitudes in women and men from adolescence to old age (Adapted from Supplemental Table 8, Rijnbeek et al. [9])

2.3 Gender Differences in Waveforms

Gender differences between 529 men and 544 women 5–96 years in age were documented by Surawicz et al. [10] for ST waveforms in chest leads, with particular attention to V2 lead. Male and female patterns were defined by J-point amplitude and ST segment slope in a 60 ms window starting at J-point. STJ amplitude ≥0.1 mV with a slope ≥20° was used to define the male pattern. The female patterns was defined by STJ <0.1 mV and apparently a slope between 0° and 20°. ST patterns not meeting these criteria were defined as indeterminate. The proportion of female pattern was high in all age groups of women and changed relatively little with age (Table 2.2). The proportion of male patterns during adolescence increased in men and there was a profound decline in the proportion of male patterns in men starting in age group 25–35 years, apparently reflecting diminishing testosterone levels with age. Sex differences in proportions of male patterns in men and female patterns in women in the report of Surawicz et al. are further highlighted in Fig. 2.4.

2.4 ST-T Waveforms in Middle-Aged Women and Men

Mean spatial vector magnitude curves ('global' ST-T wave) of the reference normal women and men free from cardiovascular disease (CVD) aged 40–65 years from the ARIC study [7] are shown in Fig. 2.5. The straight dotted lines superimposed on the

Table 2.2 Distribution of male, female, and indeterminate ECG patterns among males and females of different age groups

		Patterns in men (%)				Patterns in women (%)		
Age	No.	Male	Female	Indetemined	No.	Male	Female	Indetermined
5–7	49	63.3	32.7	4.1	60	20.0	70.0	10.0
8–12	55	54.5	38.2	7.3	52	23.1	76.9	0.0
13–16	57	80.7	15.8	3.5	57	15.8	73.7	10.5
17–24	46	91.3	6.5	2.2	47	6.4	78.7	8.5
25–35	53	73.6	11.3	15.1	51	9.8	78.4	11.8
36–45	50	58.0	24.0	18.0	50	0.0	96.0	4.0
46–54	63	47.6	42.9	9.5	68	5.9	83.8	10.3
55–75	83	30.1	54.2	15.7	83	6.0	84.3	9.6
76–96	73	13.7	69.9	16.4	76	3.9	84.2	11.8
Total	529	53.3	35.9	10.8	544	10.3	80.9	8.8

From Surawicz and Parikh [10], with permission

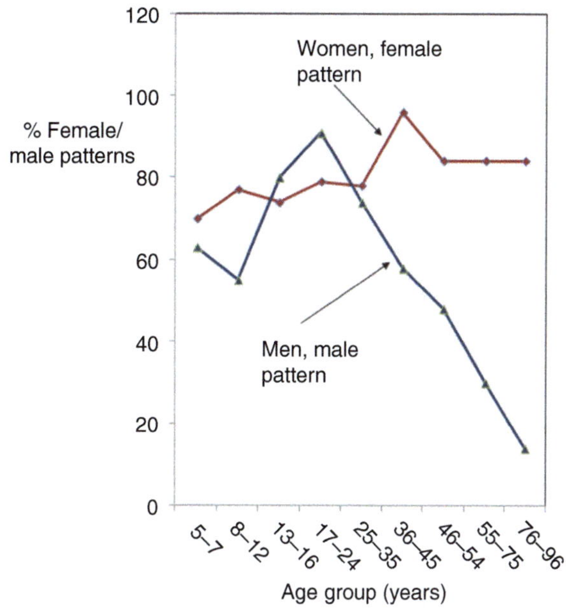

Fig. 2.4 Prevalence of male and female patterns of early ventricular repolarization in the normal ECG of males and females from childhood to old age (From Surawicz and Parikh [10], with permission)

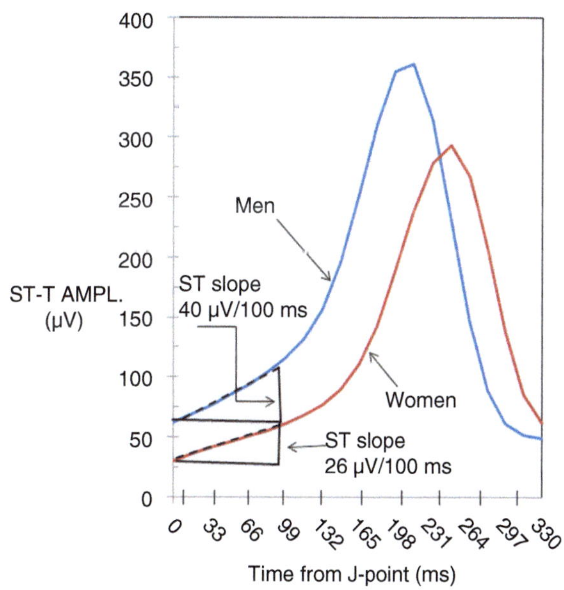

Fig. 2.5 Mean spatial vector magnitude curves ('global' ST-T wave) of the reference normal CVD-free women and men aged 40–65 years from the ARIC study [7]. The *straight dotted lines* superimposed on the initial ST segments show the ST segment slopes over the initial 100 ms of the ST segments

initial ST segments show the ST segment slopes over the initial 100 ms of the ST segments. The mean slope in women was 26 μV/100 ms increment and in men 40 μV/100 ms. The proportion of "male" and "female" ST patterns depends on the cutoff point for the slope. More detailed calculations showed that in 70 % of the men ST segment slope was 30 μV/100 ms or higher and in 65 % of the women ST segment slope was <30 μV/100 ms. Thus, with a cutoff value of 30 μV/100 ms 70 %

of men had what could be labeled as male ST pattern and 65 % of women had a female ST pattern. With cutoff for the slope at 40 μV/100 ms, 46 % of men had the "male" pattern and 85 % of the women had "female" pattern.

Direct comparison with the age-dependence of male and female patterns in the report of Suracicz et al. is difficult because slope values expressed in degrees depend on the voltage and scale and paper speed. In any case it appears that the female and male patterns are retained in the majority of middle-age women and men although the preponderance of each characteristic depends on the slope cutoff value chosen.

Detailed statistics for STJ-point amplitudes of white and African-American women 40–59 years of age are tabulated in Part 2 of this monograph, in Tables B14–B18.

2.5 Recommended Gender-Specific Criteria for ST Elevation and Depression in Standard and Monitoring Leads

The publication from the ARIC Study cited before [7] evaluated ST elevation and depression differences by gender and ethnicity in standard 12-lead ECGs and also in special monitoring leads (with RA and LA electrodes placed in subclavicular fossae and all chest lead electrodes placed at the level of V1 and V2 positions). The report contained a summary table with recommended upper limits for ST elevation and depression reproduced in Table 2.3. For ST depression in standard leads and also for monitoring leads at the level of V1 and V2 the recommended threshold values at −50 μV are uniform for all subgroups by gender and ethnicity. The recommended maximum ST elevation threshold in chest leads V2–V4 in white women (100 μV) is 50 μV lower than in white men and in African-American women (125 μV) 125 μV lower than in African-American men in whom the recommended upper normal limit is higher than in any subgroup (250 μV) in any standard or monitoring lead including the vessel-specific monitoring leads of Horaĉek [11, 12].

ST J-point elevation in white and African-American women (red columns) in two groups of chest leads is graphed in Fig. 2.6. Blue column on top of the red columns show the gender differences. Red and blue horizontal double arrows refer to the practical upper normal limits proposed in Table 2.3. The proposed upper limits for ST elevation appear reasonably valid for leads V2 and V3 and also for V1 and V5. Leads V4 and V6 fall below the limits proposed for the two lead groups. The mechanism for higher ST elevations in African-American than in white women and men is not known.

2.6 ST Segment Deviations and Sex Differences in the Risk of Cardiovascular Disease Death

Well-documented data from the Copenhagen City ECG Study demonstrate that gender differences in ST deviations carry important prognostic information for CVD mortality risk [13]. The study population, (285,194 men and women 15–90 years

Table 2.3 A summary of the threshold values[a] for ST elevation and depression in standard leads and special monitoring leads by race and sex

	White		African-American	
	Men	Women	Men	Women
ST elevation standard leads				
aVL, aVF	75	75	100	100
V2–V4	150	100	200	125
V1, V5–V6	100	75	125	100
ST Depression standard leads				
aVL, aVF	–50	–50	–75	–75
V2–V4	–50	–50	–25	–50
V1, V5–V6	–50	–50	–50	–50
ST elevation monitoring leads				
LAD	125	75	225	100
[b]MV2–MV4	150	100	200	125
LCX	50	50	75	75
[b]MaVL	100	75	175	100
[b]MV7	25	25	50	50
RCA	75	50	100	75
[b]MaVF	75	75	100	100
ST depression monitoring leads				
LAD	–50	–50	–50	–50
[b]MV2–MV4	–50	–50	–50	–50
LCX	–125	–100	–200	–100
[b]MaVL	–50	–50	–50	–50
MV7	–25	–25	–25	–25
[b]MV5	–50	–50	–25	–25
RCA	–125	–100	–175	–125
[b]MaVF	–50	–50	–50	–50

[a]Rounded to the nearest 25 μV
[b]Letter M with lead levels refers to monitoring leads *LAD* left anterior descending artery, *LCX* left circumflex artery, *RCA* right coronary artery leads

old) is a representative sample of the total population of the greater Copenhagen City. ST deviations were measured by the Marquette-GE 12-SL program at QRS offset + 1/16th of the of the average RR interval, corresponding approximately to ST segment amplitude at J-point +80 ms.

Data modified from Figs. 2.1 and 2.2 of the Copenhagen ECG Study report are listed in Table 2.4 for ST elevation and depression in leads V1 and V2 and ST depression by gender and age. The prevalence differences between men and women vary substantially by age and ST stratification level. The prevalence of ST elevation in V2 in the younger age group of women was 10 % compared to 45 % in men. As striking observation ST elevation in V2 in younger men was associated with significantly decreased risk of CVD death at all levels of ST elevation. The risk of CVD death was reduced significantly in younger women at stratification levels

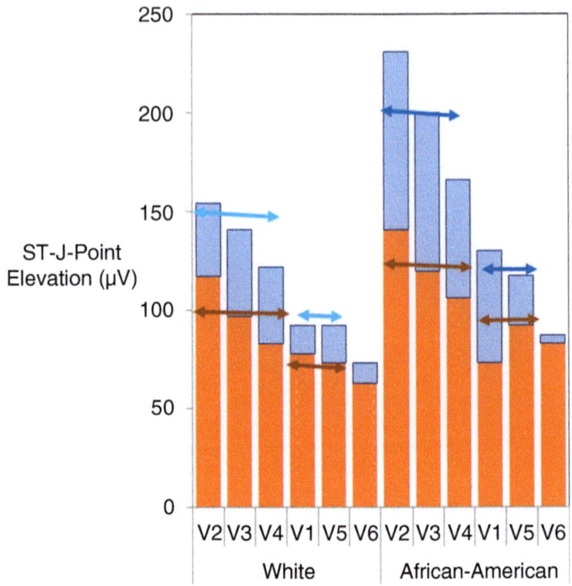

Fig. 2.6 ST J-point elevation in white and African-American women (*red columns*) in two groups of chest leads. *Blue column* on top of the *red columns* show the gender differences. *Red* and *blue horizontal double arrows* refer to the practical upper normal limits proposed in Table 2.3. The proposed upper limits seem reasonably valid for leads V2 andV3 and also for leads V1and V5. Leads V4 and V6 fall below the limits proposed for the other lead groups

Table 2.4 Prevalence of ST J-point elevation and depression exceeding 50 µV in chest leads V1 and V2 in the Copenhagen Heart Study by gender and age

Age group/ST range	Lead V1		Lead V2	
	Women	Men	Women	Men
<65 years				
>+150 µV	0.23	0.20	9.09	45.3
+100 to +150 µV	1.79	8.06	22.1	24.7
+50 to +100 µV	19.3	30.3	40.3	20.5
−50 to −100 µV	0.05	0.22	0.08	0.05
−100 to −150 µV	0	0.01	0	0.01
≤150 µV	0	0	0	0
>65 years				
>+150 µV	1.06	0.19	7.01	17.4
+100 to +150 µV	4.50	7.01	14.9	22.4
+50 to +100 µV	24.6	27.8	34.2	32.5
−50 to −100 µV	1.38	0.19	0.47	0.34
−100 to −150 µV	0.01	1.01	0.04	0.05
≤150 µV	0	0	0.01	0.01

From Rasmussen et al. [13] with permission

<150 µV. ST elevation in V1 in contrast to V2, was associated with increased risk in women and in men in both age groups at all ST levels except in younger men at ST level 50–100 µV. Consistent with previous reports, ST depression in V5 was associated with increased risk of CVD death at all ST depression levels in both age groups of women and men except in younger women at ST depression level −50 to −100 µV.

Normal limits differ in different chest leads and in men are approximately 50 μV higher than in women [3] which should be taken into consideration when comparing prevalence differences between women and men. In any case, the results from the Copenhagen n Heart Study demonstrate that ST deviation in different chest leads can be not only adverse but also favorable, reflecting at least in part differences in cardiovascular fitness. It is likely that CVD mortality risk in younger men would have been even lower if stratification by age would have been done at level lower than 65 years.

Newer risk evaluation data indicate that there is important risk information in ECG beyond that contained in the ST segment and QT interval as the data in various chapter of this monograph will show.

References

1. Davignon A, Rautaharju PM, Boisselle E, Soumis F, Megelas M, Choquette A. Normal ECG standards for infants and children. Pediatr Cardiol. 1979;1:123–31.
2. Mason JW, Ramseth DJ, Chanter DO, Moon TE, Goodman DB, Mendzelevski B. Electrocardiographic reference ranges derived from 79,743 ambulatory subjects. J Electrocardiol. 2007;40:218–34.
3. Rautaharju PM, Zhou SH, Wong S, Calhoun HP, Berenson GS, Prineas R, Davignon A. Sex differences in the evolution of the electrocardiographic QT interval with age. Can J Cardiol. 1992;8:690–5.
4. Rautaharju PM, Mason JW, Akiyama T. New age- and sex-specific criteria for QT prolongation based on rate correction formulas that minimize bias at the upper normal limits. Int J Cardiol. 2014;174(3):535–40. Erratum in: Internat J Cardiol 2014;174(x):xxx.
5. Rautaharju PM, Zhou SH, Gregg RE, Startt-Selvester RH. Electrocardiographic estimates of regional action potential durations and repolarization time subintervals reveal ischemia-induced abnormalities in acute coronary syndrome not evident from global QT. J Electrocardiol. 2011;44:718–24.
6. Rautaharju PM, Zhou SH, Gregg RE, Startt-Selvester RH. HR, gender differences, and presence versus absence of diagnostic ST elevation as determinants of spatial QRS|T angle widening in acute coronary syndrome. Am J Cardiol. 2011;107:1744–50.
7. Rautaharju PM, Zhang ZM, Haisty Jr WK, Gregg RE, Warren J, Horaĉek MB, Kucharska-Newton AM, Rosamond W, Soliman EZ. Race- and sex-associated differences in rate-adjusted QT, QTpeak, ST elevation and other regional measures of repolarization: the Atherosclerosis Risk in Communities (ARIC) Study. J Electrocardiol. 2014;47:342–50.
8. Ezaki K, Nakagava M, Tanigushi Y, Nagano Y, Teshima Y, Yufu K, Takahashi N, Nomura T, Satoh F, Mimata H, Saikawa T. Gender differences in the ST segment-effect of androgen-deprivation therapy and possible role of testosterone. Circ J. 2010;74:2448.
9. Rijnbeek PR, van Herpen G, Bots ML, Man S, Verweij N, Hofman A, Hillege H, Matthijs E, Numans ME, Swenne CA, Witteman JCM, Kors JA. Normal values of the electrocardiogram for ages 16–90 years. J Electrocardiol. 2014;47:914–21.
10. Surawicz B, Parikh SR. Prevalence of male and female patterns of early ventricular repolarization in the normal ECG of males and females from childhood to old age. J Am Coll Cardiol. 2002;40:1870–6.
11. Horácek BM, Warren JW, Penney CJ, MacLeod RS, Title LM, Gardner MJ, Feldman CL. Optimal electrocardiographic leads for detecting acute myocardial ischemia. J Electrocardiol. 2001;34(Suppl):97–111.

12. Rautaharju PM, Zhang ZM, Gregg RE, Jr Haisty WK, Vitolind MZ, Curtis AB, Warren J, Horaĉek MB, Shou SH, Soliman EZ. Normal standards for computer-ECG programs for prognostically and diagnostically important ECG variables derived from a large ethnically diverse female cohort: the Women's Health Initiative (WHI). J Electrocardiol. 2013;46:707–16.
13. Rasmussen PV, Nielsen JB, Pietersen A, Graff C, Lind B, Struijk JJ, Olesen MS, Haunsø S, Køber L, Svendsen JH, Holst AG. Electrocardiographic Precordial ST-segment deviations and the risk of cardiovascular death: results from the Copenhagen ECG Study. J Am Heart Assoc. 2014;3(3). pii: e000549. PubMed ID: 24922624.

Chapter 3
The Repolarization Model: Conceptual Considerations

Synopsis The goal of this chapter is to facilitate understanding of the repolarization model which is the backbone of this monograph. The main repolarization landmark is the peak of the T wave (Tp) on the ST-T wave spatial magnitude curve ('global' ST-T wave). At the time of Tp the largest number of left ventricular myocytes is at some point of phase 3 of their action potential. In normal repolarization sequence the time point of Tp to represent left ventricular epicardial repolarization time (RTepi). The other important landmarks of the repolarization model are Txd, the inflection point at T wave downstroke and Te, the end of the T wave, and the corresponding repolarization times (RT) RTxd and RTe. RTe is the 'global' repolarization time and RTxd is taken by the repolarization model as the best ECG estimate of endocardial repolarization time (RTendo). All RT subintervals vary with heart rate and they need to be represented as rate-adjusted intervals labeled RTea, RTpa, (RTepi)a and (RTendo)a where 'a' refers to the rate-adjusted interval. The common link between QTpa, RTepi and RTendo in the repolarization model is $\Theta(T_p|T_{ref})$, the spatial angle between Tp and Tref vectors.

A rhombic lattice dividing space into 12 equal-sized directions is used to quantify three-dimensional (3-D) spatial distributions of repolarization vectors. A display format is introduced for practical display of 3-D data as a 2-D display obtained by opening up the 3-D rhombic lattice in posterior midline and projecting all 12 rhombic faces to the frontal plane. In this display the majority of Tp vectors (66 %) in normal women are in direction Inferior-Left-Anterior (ILA), with 22 % in direction Left (L) and 10 % in Anterior-Left (AL) as the faces of the rhombus are labeled in order of the spatial directional dominance with respect to principal axes. Because the spatial direction of repolarization is diametrically opposite to the direction of the Tp vector, the normal direction of repolarization sequence is in 66 % of the women in Superior-Right-Posterior (SRP), 22 % in Right (R) and 10 % in Posterior-Left (PL) direction. This indicates a relatively tight directional clustering of normal repolarization.

P.M. Rautaharju, *The Female Electrocardiogram: Special Repolarization Features, Gender Differences, and the Risk of Adverse Cardiac Events*,
DOI 10.1007/978-3-319-15293-6_3

Abbreviations and Symbols

AL	Anterior-left
ILA	Inferior-left-anterior
L	Left
PR	Posterior-right
QTe	QTend interval
RT	Repolarization time
RTe	'Global' repolarization time (equal to QTe)
RTea	Rate-adjusted RTe
RTendo	Endocardial repolarization time
(RTendo)a	Rate-adjusted RTendo
RTepi	Epicardial repolarization time
(RTepi)a	Rate-adjusted RTepi
RTp	RTpeak interval
SRP	Superior-right-posterior
Tp	Peak of the global T wave

3.1 Temporal Landmarks of Repolarization

The main ECG variables from the repolarization model are defined in Table 3.1. The landmarks of repolarization are labeled on the graph of the ST-T wave magnitude curve (the global T wave) in Fig. 3.1. The main repolarization landmark is the peak of the T wave (Tp). At the time of Tp the largest number of left ventricular myocytes is at some point of phase 3 of their action potential. RTp in Fig. 3.1 denotes repolarization time (RT) of the left ventricular myocyte layers which in normal repolarization reach the end of their repolarization at time of Tp. The other important global T wave landmarks are To, the onset of the T wave, and Txd, the inflection point at T wave downstroke and Te, the end of the T wave. In addition to RTp, the other two important repolarization times in the model are RTxd and RTe. RTe corresponds to the QTe interval and RTxd is the QTxd interval. RTxd is taken by the repolarization model as the best ECG estimate of endocardial repolarization time (RTendo).

3.2 Two-Dimensional Reference Frame for Quantization of Three-Dimensional Distributions of ECG Variables

Electrophysiologists generally consider the time point of Tp to represent left ventricular epicardial repolarization (RTepi). However, as shown next this assertion is valid only if Tp vector direction is normal, i.e., if the spatial direction of repolarization sequence is normal. Thus, it is necessary to consider spatial direction of

Table 3.1 Definitions of main ECG variables of the repolarization model

Acronym	Description	Excel algorithm
QT_{pa}	Rate adjusted QT_p Interval (ms)	Log-linear formulas:
		$QTpa = QTp - 295 * (RR^{0.40} - 1)$ *for men,*
		$QTpa = 303 * (RR^{0.40} - 1)$ *for women*
		Alternative linear formulas:
		$QT_{pa} = QT_p + 121 * (1 - RR)$ *for men,*
		$QT_{pa} = QT_e + 113 * (1 - RR)$ *for women.*
T_pT_{xd}	LV crossmural repolarization time gradient (ms)	T_pT_{xd} = interval from T_p to T_{xd}, where T_{xd} is the inflection point at global T wave downstroke
RT_{epi}	Epicardial repolarization time (ms)	$RT_{epi} = QT_{pa} - (\text{Cos}\theta(T_p \mid T_{ref}) - 1) * T_pT_{xd} / 2$
RT_{xd} = RTendo	LV repolarization time at time point T_{xd} (ms)	$RT_{xd} = QT_{pa} + (\text{Cos}\theta(T_p \mid T_{ref}) + 1) * T_pT_{xd} / 2$
$^a\Theta(T_p \vert T_{ref})$	Tp vector deviation angle from normal reference direction (°)	$\theta(T_p \mid T_{ref}) = 57.3 * \text{ACOS}(T_pX * T_{ref}X + T_pY * T_{ref}Y + T_pZ * T_{ref}Z) / (T_pV * T_{ref}V)$
$\Theta(R \vert STT)$	Spatial angle between the mean QRS and STT vectors	$\theta(Rm \mid STTm) = 57.3 * \text{ACOS}(RmX * STT_mX + R_mY * STT_mY + R_mZ * STT_mZ) / (R_mV * STT_mV)$
$\Theta(R_p \vert T_p)$	Spatial angle between the peak QRS and T vectors	$\theta(Rp_{\vert}T_p) = 57.3 * \text{ACOS}(R_pX * TpX + R_pY * T_pY + R_pZ * T_pZ) / (R_pV * T_pV)$
$\Theta(T_{init} \vert T_{term})$	Spatial angle between the mean initial and terminal T vectors	$\theta(T_{init} \mid T_{term}) = 57.3 * \text{ACOS}(T_{init}X * T_{term}X + T_{init}Y * T_{term}Y + T_{init}Z * T_{term}Z) / (T_{init}V * T_{init}V)$
$\Theta(T_{term} \vert T_{ref})$	Spatial angle between the mean terminal T vector and Tref vector	$\theta(T_{term} \mid T_{ref}) = 57.3 * \text{ACOS}(T_{term}X * T_{ref}X + T_{term}Y * T_{ref}Y + T_{term}Z * T_{ref}Z) / (T_{term}V * T_{ref}V)$

LV denotes left ventricle; Symbol * denotes multiplication sign

V in the algorithms refers to spatial vector magnitude and ACOS to archcosine

$\Theta(T_{init}|T_{term})$ is the spatial angle between the mean initial and terminal T vectors from quintiles 1 to 3 and 4 to 5 of repolarization, respectively

$^a\Theta(T_p|T_{ref})$ is the spatial angle between Tp and Tref vectors and $T_{ref}X$, $T_{ref}Y$, $T_{ref}Z$ are the xX, Y and Z components of the normal T reference vector (T_{ref}) with unit vector components(0.741, 0.563, –0.367) in women and (0.626, 0.463, –0.627) in men

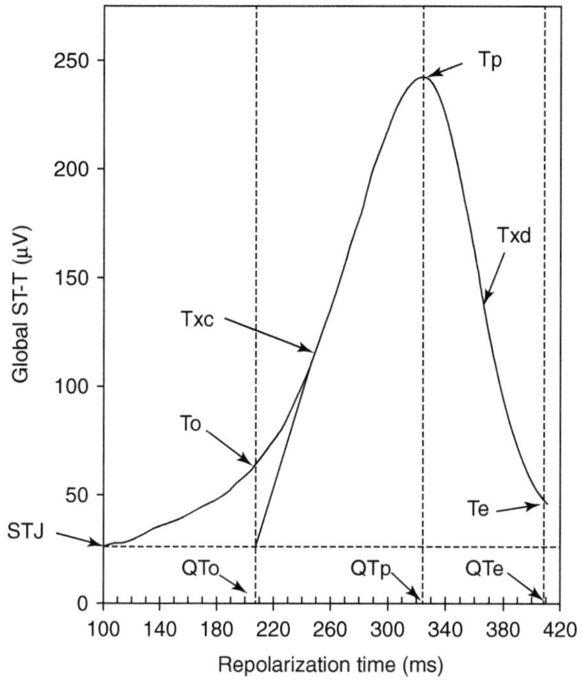

Fig. 3.1 A schematic illustrating main variables of the repolarization model defined explicitly in Table 3.1. In normal repolarization sequence, RTp represents RTepi. The TpTe interval is a measure of global temporal RT gradient or global RT dispersion, and the TpTxd interval is the regional left ventricular free wall cross-mural RT gradient (XMRTgrad). A line extrapolated backward to the intersection of the *horizontal line* from the end of QRS identified time point of To. Te is T wave end; To T wave onset; Txc inflexion point (maximum slope) at T wave upstroke; and Txd is the Inflexion point (minimum slope) at T wave downstroke. STT vector magnitude curve is shown at 40 sample points along RT from QRS end to Te. *Arrows* at RTp, RTxd, and RTend indicate RT at point of Tp, Txd, and Te, respectively

repolarization at time point of Tp in order to properly estimate RTepi and RTendo. A rhombic lattice dividing space into 12 equal-sized directions is used to quantify spatial distributions of repolarization vectors (Fig. 3.2). A practical display of 3-D distributions is shown for RTp in normal women in Fig. 3.3. This display is obtained by opening up the 3-D rhombic lattice in posterior midline and projecting all 12 rhombic faces to the frontal plane such as shown in Sect. 3.4.

3.3 Functional Relationships Between QTpa, RTepi and RTendo

The common link between QTpa, RTepi and RTendo in the repolarization model is $\Theta(T_p \mid T_{ref})$, the spatial angle between Tp and Tref vectors where Tref is the unit reference vector for spatial direction of Tp vector in normal repolarization. The x, y and z components of this unit vector (spatial magnitude = 1) in women are (0.741,

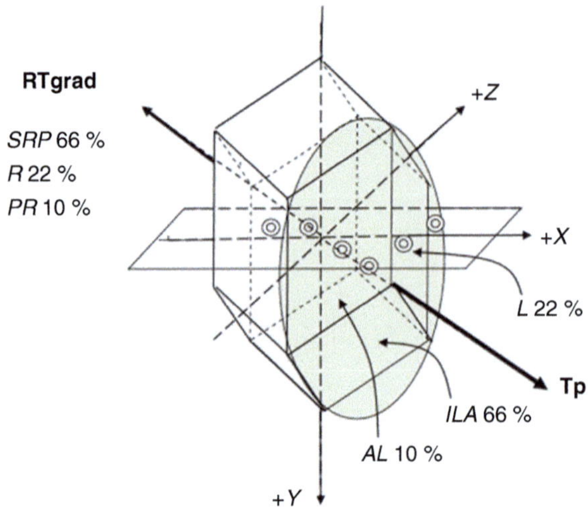

Fig. 3.2 Anterior view of a rhombic duododecahedron lattice with 12 symmetrical spatial reference directions used for quantifying directional distributions of ECG vectors. The letters in the acronyms denote the directions in order of the closeness to left (*L*), right (*R*), inferior (*I*), superior (*S*), anterior (*A*) and posterior (*P*) directions of the X, Y and Z axis. In normal repolarization 96 % of the Tpeak (Tp) vectors are within the *oval shaded light orange* in reference directions left, inferior-left-anterior and anterior-left (*L*, *ILA* and *AL*, respectively)

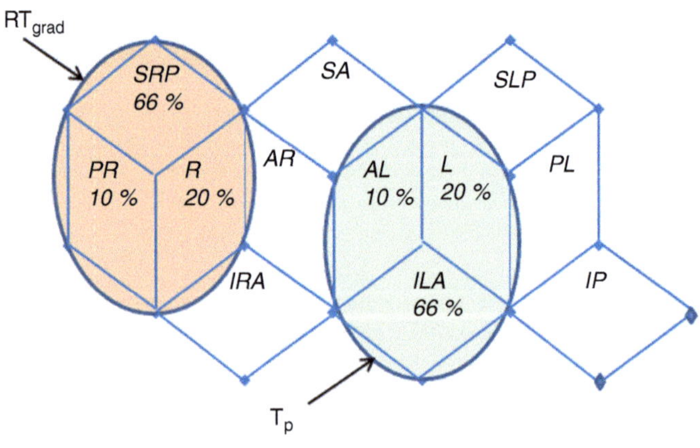

Fig. 3.3 Distribution of Tpeak (Tp) vector and repolarization time gradient (RTgrad) vectors in 12 spatial directions in normal adult women in simplified representation of the 3-D display in Fig. 3.2. The 3-D rhombus was opened at posterior midline and the rhombic faces were projected on the frontal plane. The letters in the labels refer to the six principal directions: *L* Left, *R* Right, *I* Inferior, *S* Superior, *A* Anterior, *P* Posterior. The letters in acronyms for rhombic faces are in order of dominance of principal axis: *ILA* Inferior-Left-Anterior, etc. Spatial distribution of the RTgrad vectors is diametrically opposite to Tp vector distribution because current flow during repolarization is opposite to that during depolarization

0.563, –0.367). These coordinates define the spatially tightly clustered direction of normal repolarization.

As defined in Table 3.1, $\text{RTepi} = \text{QT}_{pa} - \left(\text{Cos}\theta\left(\text{T}_p \mid \text{T}_{ref}\right) - 1\right) * \text{T}_p\text{T}_{xd} / 2$. Thus, RTepi is obtained by subtracting from RTepi the modifying term $\left(\text{Cos}\theta\left(\text{T}_p \mid \text{T}_{ref}\right) - 1\right) * \text{T}_p\text{T}_{xd} / 2$. In normal repolarization the spatial angle is small, <30° and $\text{Cos}\theta\left(\text{T}_p \mid \text{T}_{ref}\right)$ does not differ much from 1. Thus, the correction term is small and $\text{RTepi} = \text{QTpa}$. In conditions such as left bundle branch block (LBBB) and ECG pattern of left ventricular strain in left ventricular hypertrophy (LVH), $\theta\left(\text{T}_p \mid \text{T}_{ref}\right)$ is close to 180° and cosine between T_p and T_{ref} vectors is close to –1 and the term $\left(\text{Cos}\theta\left(\text{T}_p \mid \text{T}_{ref}\right) - 1\right)$ is close to –2. The mean value of TpTxd interval in normal women being 40 ms means that $\text{RTepi} = \text{QTpa} - 40\,\text{ms}$. Similarly, $\text{RTendo} = \text{QTpa} + 40$ because $\text{RTendo} = \text{QT}_{pa} + \left(\text{Cos}\theta\left(\text{T}_p \mid \text{T}_{ref}\right) + 1\right) * \text{T}_p\text{T}_{xd} / 2$ as defined in Table 3.1. This implies that the direction of left ventricular lateral wall repolarization has become concordant with respect to excitation and repolarization occurs from endocardial to epicardial direction.

In case the site of the earliest repolarization shifts from the lateral wall to anterior wall epicardium with shortening of epicardial action potential durations in ischemia induced by left anterior descending artery narrowing, the direction of repolarization becomes near perpendicular to the Tref direction. Assuming a shift of 90° in Tp vector direction, $\text{Cos}\theta\left(\text{T}_p \mid \text{T}_{ref}\right) = 0$ and $\left(\text{Cos}\theta\left(\text{T}_p \mid \text{T}_{ref}\right) - 1\right) = -1$. This implies that $\text{RTepi} = \text{QTpa} - 20\,\text{ms}$ and $\text{RTendo} = \text{QTpa} + 20$, so that $\text{RTepi} = \text{RTendo}$ and repolarization in the lateral wall proceeds perpendicular Tref and parallel to epicardium and endocardium.

3.4 Relationship Between T Peak Vectors and Spatial Direction of Repolarization Sequence

Figure 3.3 shows that the majority of Tp vectors (66 %) in normal women are in direction Inferior-Left-Posterior (ILP), with 22 % in direction Left (L) and 10 % in Anterior-Left (AL) as the faces of the rhombus are labeled in Fig. 3.3. Consequently, the normal direction of repolarization sequence is in 66 % in direction Superior-Right-Posterior (SRP), 22 % in Right (R) and 10 % in Posterior-Left (PL) direction. While the directions of the QRS vectors and depolarization sequence are identical, spatial direction of repolarization sequence generating the T wave is diametrically opposite to T vector directions because repolarization currents flow is in direction opposite to that of excitation currents (Tables 3.2, 3.3 and 3.4).

Table 3.2 Mean values, standard deviations and normal 2nd to 98th percentile range for main parameters of the repolarization model

	White		African-American		P for racial difference	
	Men	Women	Men	Women	Men	Women
[a]RT_{epi} (ms)	314; 14.9	331; 15.7	310;17.6	330; 18.7	0.001	0.327
	285→345	300→365	280→345	295→365		
[a]RT_{endo} (ms)	347; 15.2	362; 15.8	343;17.1	362; 18.9	0.001	0.412
	320→380	330→395	310→380	325→405		
[b]APD_{epi} (ms)	273; 15.8	290; 16.5	269;18.5	289; 19.2	0.001	0.871
	240→305	255→325	235→305	255→330		
[b]APD_{endo} (ms)	337; 15.2	352; 15.8	333;17.1	252; 18.9	0.001	0.024
	310→370	320→385	300→370	320→395		
[c]QR_p (ms)	41; 5.4	41; 5.6	41; 5.3	41; 5.4	0.019	0.024
	30→55	30→55	30→55	30→55		
[d]RNDPV(μV)	50; 19.6	41; 15.7	67; 27.9	46; 18.9	0.001	0.001
	20→100	20→85	30→135	20→95		
[e]$\Theta(R_m\|STT_m)$	56; 26.2	47; 24.9	64; 28.2	52; 28.8	0.001	0.001
	15→120	10→105	20→140	10→135		
[f]$\Theta(R_m\| T_m)$	56; 24.1	46; 21.8	59; 24.6	42; 22.6	0.001	0.001
	15→110	10→100	15→115	5→100		
[g]$\Theta(R_p\|T_p)$	48; 28.8	38; 26.5	61; 34.2	45; 32.1	0.001	0.170
	10→135	5→110	15→155	5→145		
[h]$\Theta(T_p\|T_{ref})$	17; 10.6	15; 10.2	21; 14.0	18; 13.8	0.001	0.001
	5→45	0→40	5→60	5→55		
[i]$\Theta(T_{term}\|T_{ref})$	19; 12.3	17; 12.1	28; 19.4	25; 21.8	0.001	0.001
	5→50	0→50	5→90	5→100		
[j]$\Theta(T_{init}\|T_{erm})$	17; 10.6	15; 10.2	21; 14.0	18; 13.8	0.001	0.001
	5→45	0→40	5→60	10→50		

(continued)

Table 3.2 (continued)

	White		African-American		P for racial difference	
	Men	Women	Men	Women	Men	Women
[l]ST_oV (μV)	49; 23.1	32; 16.5	78; 29.8	47; 21.8	0.001	0.001
	10→100	5→75	25→145	10→100		
[l]T_oV (μV)	144; 51.7	100; 37.6	188;57.2	120; 45.3	0.001	0.001
	55→260	35→190	75→310	45→220		
[l]T_pV (μV)	403; 137.3	327; 118.8	424; 141	312; 130.6	0.001	0.001
	155→725	115→595	160→720	100→610		
[m]T_oV/T_pV	36;7.0	32; 8.1	46; 9.4	40; 10.6	0.001	0.001
(%)	25→50	20→55	30→70	25→70		

From Rautaharju et al. [1]

P for significance of the sex difference of the mean values was <0.001 for all variables in white men and women except $p=0.084$ for $\Theta(T_p|T_{ref})$ and for all variables in African-American men and women except $p=0.078$ for $\Theta(T_p|T_{ref})$, $p=0.315$ for $\Theta(T_p|T_{ref})$ and $p=0.010$ for $\Theta(T_{term}|T_{ref})$

Intervals rounded to nearest 5 ms, angles to nearest 5° and amplitudes to nearest 5 μV

[a]RT_{epi} = ECG estimate of subepicardial repolarization time (RT_{epi}) and RT_{endo} =ECG estimate of subendocardial repolarization time (RT_{endo})

[b]APD_{epi} and APD_{endo} = epicardial and endocardial action potential duration, respectively

[c]QR_p = interval from QRS onset to the peak of the global T wave

[d]RNDPV = nondipolar QRS and TNDPV = nondipolar T wave components (square roots of the total variance of components 4–8 from singular value decomposition)

[e]$\Theta(R_m|STT_m)$ = spatial angle between the mean QRS and STT vectors

[f]$\Theta(R_m|T_m)$ = spatial angle between the mean QRS and T vectors

[g]$\Theta(R_p|T_p)$ = spatial angle between the peak QRS and T vectors

[h]$\Theta(T_p|T_{ref})$ = spatial angle between the Tp vector and the reference T vector (Tref), signifying spatial deviation angle of repolarization direction from the direction of the normal repolarization sequence

[i]$\Theta(T_{term}|T_{ref})$ = spatial angle between the mean terminal T vector and Tref vector

[j]$\Theta(T_{init}|T_{erm})$ = spatial angle between the mean initial and terminal T vectors from quintiles 1 to 3 and quintiles 4 to 5 of global T wave, respectively

[k]T wave complexity = average ratio of the second and the first eigenvalue from singular value decomposition

[l]Symbol 'V' with ST_oV, T_oV and T_pV signifies vector magnitude of ST_o, T_o and T_p, respectively

[m]T_oV/T_pV = the ratio of T onset and T peak vector magnitudes

Table 3.3 Definitions of key electrocardiographic variables used in the repolarization model

Accronym	Description	Excel algorithm
QT_{pa}	Rate adjusted QT_p Interval (ms)	$QT_{pa} = QT_p + 121 * (1 - RR)$ for men,
		$QT_{pa} = QT_e + 113 * (1 - RR)$ for women.
T_pT_{xd}	LV crossmural repolarization time gradient (ms)	T_pT_{xd} = interval from T_p to T_{xd}, where T_{xd} is the inflection point at global T wave downstroke
RTepi	Epicardial repolarization time (ms)	$RT_{epi} = QT_{pa} - (Cos\theta(T_p \mid T_{ref}) - 1) * T_pT_{xd} / 2$
RT_{xd}	LV repolarization time at time point T_{xd} (ms)	$RT_{xd} = QT_{pa} + (Cos\theta(T_{init} \mid T_{ref}) + 1) * T_pT_{xd} / 2$
$\Theta(T_p \mid T_{ref})$	Tp vector deviation angle from normal reference direction (°)	$\theta(T_p \mid T_{ref}) = 57.3 * ACOS(T_pX * T_{ref}x + T_pY * T_{ref}y + T_pZ * T_{ref}z) / (T_pV * T_{ref}V)$†
$\Theta(R \mid STT)$	Spatial angle between the mean QRS and STT vectors.	$\theta(R_m \mid STT_m) = 57.3 * ACOS(R_mX * STT_mX + R_mY * STT_mY + R_mZ * STT_mZ) / (R_mV * STT_mV)$
$\Theta(R_p \mid T_p)$	Spatial angle between the peak QRS and T vectors	$\theta(Rp_{\mid}T_p) = 57.3 * ACOS(R_pX * TpX + R_pY * T_pY + R_pZ * T_pZ) / (R_pV * T_pV)$
$\Theta(T_{init} \mid T_{term})$	Spatial angle between the mean initial and terminal T vectors	$\theta(T_{init} \mid T_{term}) = 57.3 * ACOS(T_{init}X * T_{term}X + T_{init}Y * T_{term}Y + T_{init}Z * T_{term}Z) / (T_{init}V * T_{init}V)$
$\Theta(T_{term} \mid T_{ref})$	Spatial angle between the mean terminal T vector and Tref vector	$\theta(T_{term} \mid T_{ref}) = 57.3 * ACOS(T_{term}X * T_{ref}x + T_{term}Y * T_{ref}y + T_{term}Z * T_{ref}z) / (T_{term}V * T_{ref}V)$

LV denotes left ventricle; Symbol * denotes multiplication sign
V in the algorithms refers to spatial vector magnitude and ACOS to archcosine
$T_{ref}x$, $T_{ref}y$, $T_{ref}z$ are the x,y and z components of the normal T reference vector (T_{ref}) with unit vector xyz components (0.695, 0.537, –0.478)

Table 3.4 Unit xyz components for 12 spatial reference directions of the rhombic duododecahedron

Label	Direction[a]	x	y	z
L	Left	1	0	0
ILA	Inferior-left-anterior	0.497	0.819	−0.287
AL	Anterior-left	0.5	0	−0.866
SA	Superior-anterior	0	−0.819	−0.574
AR	Anterior-right	−0.5	0	−0.866
IRA	Inferior-right-anterior	−0.497	0.819	−0.287
R	Right	−1	0	0
SRP	Superior-right-posterior	−0.497	−0.819	0.287
PR	Posterior-right	−0.5	0	0.866
IP	Inferior-posterior	0	0.819	0.574
PL	Posterior-left	0.5	0	0.866
SLP	Superior-left-posterior	0.497	−0.819	0.287

[a]Spatial directions in order of closeness to principal six directions

Reference

1. Rautaharju PM, Zhang ZM, Warren J, Haisty WK, Prineas RJ, Kurcharska-Newton AM, Rosamond WD, Soliman EZ. Electrocardiographic predictors of coronary heart disease and sudden cardiac deaths in men and women free from cardiovascular disease in the Atherosclerosis Risk in Communities (ARIC) Study. J Am Heart Assoc. 2013;2(3):e000061. doi:10.1161/JAHA.113.000061.

Chapter 4
Electrocardiographic Predictors Coronary Heart Disease Death

Synopsis In many industrialized countries including the US cardiovascular disease (CVD) continues to be the leading cause of death. Women have been increasingly included in CVD intervention efforts but substantial gender differences still remain in CVD prevalence and mortality. Annual number of adults with diagnosed heart attack of fatal coronary heart disease (CHD) occurs 10 years later in women than in men. Differences in population demographics account for the fact that in terms of absolute numbers more women are living with and dying from CVD including stroke than men, and more women than men are discharged from hospitals with diagnosis heart failure and stroke. These facts emphasize the need for identification of improved ECG predictors for CVD death and HF.

In the WHI study in post-menopausal women the main independent predictors of CHD death were $\Theta(T_{p|}T_{ref})$, the spatial angle between the Tpeak (Tp) vector and the reference vector for normal repolarization (Rfef) and TaVR amplitude, with an over twofold increased risk for both. $\Theta(T_{p|}T_{ref})$ is the spatial angle between the T peak vector and the normal T reference vector. In the ARIC study in CVD-free middle-aged men and women, the spatial angle between the mean QRS and Tvectors, $[\Theta(R_m|T_m)]$ was the strongest independent predictor of CHD death with over twofold increased risk in women and 1.4-fold increased risk in men. $\Theta(T_{p|}T_{ref})$ was also an independent predictor of CHD death, with 1.7-fold increased risk. TV1amplitude was an additional independent predictor in women with a twofold increased risk and TaVR amplitude and the rate-adjusted QT interval were additional independent predictors in men, with an approximately 50 % increased risk.

$\Theta(T_{p|}T_{ref})$ angle was consistently a strong independent predictor for CHD death. This spatial angle is a measure of deviant direction of the spatial repolarization sequence from the direction of normal repolarization approximately in the direction of the axis of lead aVR. Widened $\Theta(T_{p|}T_{ref})$ angle commonly occurs with anterior-right rotation of the Tp vector. TaVR and also TV1 can thus be expected to be sensitive indicators of deviant direction of repolarization. TaVR is functionally dependent on $\Theta(T_{p|}T_{ref})$ angle and both can be considered as primary alternative choices as independent predictors of CHD death. The simplicity of aVR makes it a particularly attractive choice in practical clinical applications.

P.M. Rautaharju, *The Female Electrocardiogram: Special Repolarization Features, Gender Differences, and the Risk of Adverse Cardiac Events*,
DOI 10.1007/978-3-319-15293-6_4

Abbreviations and Acronyms

AHA	American Heart Association
ARIC	Arteriosclerosis research in communities
CHD	Coronary heart disease
CV	Cornell voltage
CVD	Cardiovascular disease
MRFIT	Mutiple risk factor intervention trial
ToV/TpV	Ratio of T vectors at time points of the onset and peak of the T wave vector magnitude function
WHI	Women's health initiative
Θ(Rm|STTm)	Spatial angle between the mean QRS and ST-T vectors
Θ(Rm|Tm)	Spatial angle between the mean QRS and T vectors
Θ(Tinit|Tterm)	Spatial angle between the initial and terminal T vectors from repolarization quintiles 1 to 3 and 4 to 5, respectively
Θ(Tp|Tref)	Spatial angle between Tpeak (Tp)vector and tne normal reference T vector (Tref)

4.1 Introduction

Early epidemiological studies on coronary heart disease (CHD) focused almost exclusively on men. CHD was considered a male disease and major epidemiological studies such as the Seven Countries' Study [1] and major clinical trials such as the Multiple Risk Factor Intervention Trial (MRFIT) [2] involved men only. Women's health issues had a low priority in medical research until after 1985 when Federal and American Heart Association (AHA) launched initiatives to reduce gender disparities in research and clinical care. Political pressure gradually changed the situation and as a result major research programs including women were introduced such as the large-scale Women's Health Initiative (WHI) study in 1991 [3].

In spite of intervention efforts, cardiovascular disease (CVD) continues to be the leading killer in the US and substantial sex differences still remain in CVD prevalence and mortality. In terms of absolute numbers, more women are living with and dying from CVD including stroke than men and more women than men are discharged from hospitals with diagnosis heart failure and stroke [4]. This is due to differences in population demographics with a larger proportion of women than men in elderly population groups where CVD prevalence is highest. However, the prevalence of and the mortality from CHD in each stratum of age is higher in men than in women until after 75 years of age as shown in Fig. 4.1a from Mosca et al. [4]. As the authors comment, this may have contributed to the perception that heart disease is man's disease. A closer examination of Fig. 4.1 of Mosca et al. shows that CHD events in men occur approximately at 10 years younger age than in women. This is apparent from Fig. 4.1b where the age strata in women are shifter by 10 years.

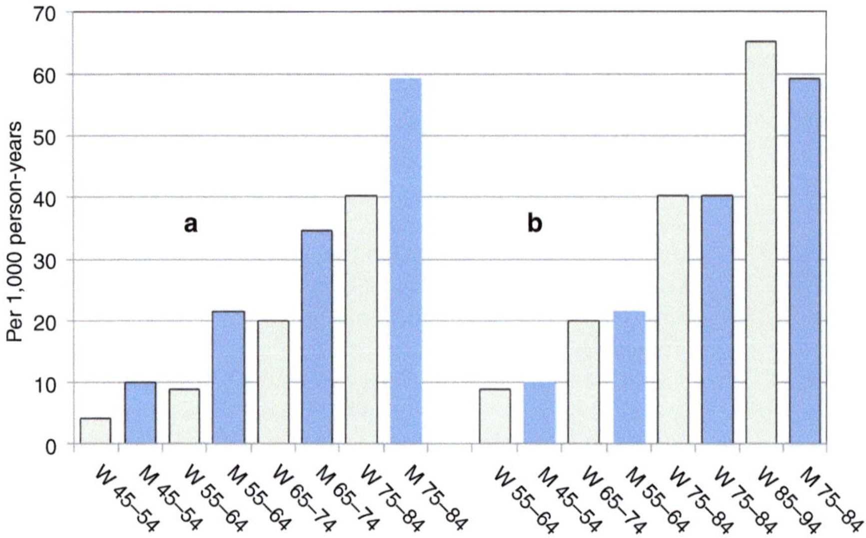

Fig. 4.1 Annual number of adults having diagnosed heart attack or fatal coronary heart disease in men (*M*) and women (*W*) (**a**), and with age groups of women shifted by 10 years compared to men (**b**) (Modified from Mosca et al. [4], with permission)

Mosca et al. also comment on a statistically significant trend in CHD mortality rates among younger women 35–44 years of age which were found to have increased an average of 1.3 % annually between 1997 and 2002 [5].

4.2 QRS and ST-T Variables as Predictors of Coronary Heart Disease Death in Post-menopausal Women

Table 4.1 lists hazard ratios for QRS and ST-T variables which were significant predictors for CHD death from an early report from the WHI study with a 9.2 year follow-up [6]. Two of the significant CHD mortality predictors, Cornell voltage and rate-adjusted QT interval had a significant interaction with CVD status at baseline. Hazard ratios for these two variables are listed separately for CVD-Free and CVD groups, and hazard ratios for the rest of the significant ECG predictors are listed for the combined group. In this study, the cut-off point selected at 95th percentile of the normal reference group which for instance for the Cornell-voltage (CV) was 1,800 μV. This cut-off point is lower than the commonly used the upper normal limit for CV (2,000 μV). The table lists hazard ratios for multivariable-adjusted single variable models and for multivariable-adjusted multiple ECG variable models. The ECG variables chosen by the multivariable model were selected by a reverse selection procedure from a set of variables with low correlations. The variables remaining in these models can be considered as independent predictors of CHD mortality.

Table 4.1 Hazard ratios (95 % confidence intervals) for ECG predictors of CHD death in WHI women by CVD status at baseline

	[a]Multivariable-adjusted single ECG variable models		[a]Multivariable-adjusted multiple ECG variable models	
ECG variable (95 % cutpoint from reference group)	CVD-free group	CVD group	CVD-free group	CVD group
‡QTrr				
Reference (<437 ms)	1	1	1	1
Prolonged (≥437 ms)	2.17 (1.24–3.73)**	0.47 (0.14–1.54)	1.90 (1.09–3.33)*	0.45 (0.14–1.50)
§Cornell voltage				
Reference (<1,800 μV)	1	1	1	1
High (≥1,800 μV)	1.91 (1.09–1.36)	0.48 (0.17–1.37)	1.25 (0.69–2.26)	0.36 (0.12–1.05)
	CVD-free and CVD groups combined		CVD-free and CVD groups combined	
‖Θ(Rm|Tm)				
Reference (<56°)	1		1	
Borderline (57–96°)	1.32 (0.85–2.04)		1.23 (0.79–1.93)	
Wide (≥97°)	2.70 (1.65–4.39)***		2.12 (1.23–3.62)**	
#ECG MI/ischemic injury				
No	1		1	
Yes	2.41 (1.52–3.81)***		1.87 (1.15–3.03)*	
††QRS non-dipolar voltage				
Reference (<65 μV)	1		1	
Increased (≥65 μV)	2.18 (1.33–3.57)**		1.85 (1.11–3.08)*	
TV5 mean amplitude				
Normal (73–235 μV)	1		Removed in backward selection	
Low (<73 μV); (Tpeak <117 μV)	1.80 (1.16–2.81)**			
STV5 mean amplitude				
Reference (>0 μV)	1		Removed in backward selection	
Depressed (≤0 μV)	1.63 (1.07–2.47)*			

Modified from Rautaharju et al. [6]
CHD coronary heart disease, *CVD* cardiovascular disease, *WHI* Women's Health Initiative
Symbols *, ** and *** signify P values <0.05, <0.01 and <0.001, respectively, for hazard ratios
[a]Each ECG variable was evaluated individually in single-variable models and variables in multiple ECG variable models were selected by a backward-selection procedure to identify independent predictors. Both models were adjusted for age, ethnicity, systolic blood pressure, and body mass index and the following clinical and therapeutic variables: smoking, hormone therapy use at baseline, self-report of the use of cholesterol-lowering drugs, self-report of diabetes control, or the use of cardioactive drugs (antiarrhythmic drugs, calcium channel blockers, β-blockers, diuretics, antidepressants, or psychotherapeutic drugs)
‡QTrr is QT rate-adjusted as a linear function of the RR interval; §Cornell voltage = RV5 + DV3; ‖Θ(Rm|Tm) is the spatial angle between the mean QRS and T vectors; #ECG MI/ischemic injury as defined by the Cardiac Injury Score; †† QRS non-dipolar voltage from singular value decomposition

The strongest predictors of CHD mortality in multivariable-adjusted single ECG variable models in women with CVD and CVD-free groups combined were the spatial angle between the mean QRS and T vectors ($\Theta(R_m|T_m)$) and old myocardial infarct by ECG (ECG-MI), with 2.70-fold increased risk for $\Theta(R_m|T_m)$ and 2.14-fold increased risk for ECG-MI. The risk for high QRS nondipolar voltage was also increased over twofold. CHD mortality risk for rate adjusted QT was increased significantly, 2.17-fold, only in CVD-free women ($P<0.01$). Rate adjustment for QT in that 2006 report was done as a linear function of the RR interval whereby in women QTrr = QT-0.185*(RR-1), with QT and RR in seconds [7].

Among the ECG variables identified as independent predictors, wide $\Theta(R_m|T_m)$ was associated with a 2.12-fold increased risk of CHD death, and the risk increase for old myocardial infarction (MI) by ECG (ECG-MI) was1.87-fold, 1.85-fold for QRS nondipolar voltage and 1.90-fold for rate -adjusted QT (for the latter variable in CVD-free group only).

4.3 Repolarization-Related Variables as Predictors of Coronary Heart Disease Death in Post-menopausal Women

4.3.1 ECG Predictors Evaluated as Single Variables in Women

A recent WHI report evaluated the risk for CHD death for ECG variables from the repolarization model in 52,994 women from a longer follow-up period (average 16.9 years) during which 941 CHD deaths occurred [8]. The study group was stratified by CVD status at baseline. Selection criteria for participants considered to have CVD (N=12,569) included history of angina pectoris, coronary bypass operation, and congestive heart failure. In addition, from the group of women initially classified as CVD-free, those with silent ECG-MI, AF or ECG-LVH (Cornell voltage >1,200 μV combined with Minnesota Code 4.1–4.3) or ischemic ST depression (isolated Minnesota Code 4.1–4.2) were transferred to the CVD group, leaving 52,092 women into the CVD-free group.

A large number of ECG variables were significant predictors of CHD death when evaluated as single ECG variables even after multivariable-adjustment for demographic/clinical factors (Table 4.2). The strongest predictors of CHD death in CVD-free women were heart rate, Θ(Rm|Tm), Θ(Tp|Tref), Tampl.V6 and ToV/TpV, with an over 1.5-fold increase in risk for each. The risk was nearly twofold for ToV/TpV (the ratio of T onset and T peak vector magnitudes (ToV and TpV, respectively)) of the ST-T spatial magnitude curve at time points To and Tp. A high ToV/TpV ratio reflects reduced convexity or triangularization of the action potentials of the left lateral wall myocytes. As in CVD-free women, a large number of ECG variables including ToV/TpV in women with CVD were strong predictors of CHD death when evaluated as single ECG variables. The risk for CHD death was increased over-1.5-fold for 12 ECG variables and over twofold increase for two of them, $\Theta(T_p|T_{ref})$ and STJV6.

Table 4.2 Single ECG variable multivariable-adjusted hazard ratios with 95 % confidence intervals for CHD death in women by CVD status at baseline

	CVD-free group				CVD group			
	Test quintile	Limit[a]	HR (95 % CI)[b]	P value	Test quintile	Limit[a]	HR (95 % CI)[b]	P value
Heart rate	Q5	>74	1.51 (1.28–1.79)	<0.0001	Q5	>74	1.37 (1.12–1.68)	0.0022
[c]QT_{ea} (ms)	Q5	>425	1.25 (1.07–1.49)	0.0077	Q5	>428	1.23 (1.00–1.51)	0.0468
[c]QT_{pa} (ms)	Q5	>354	1.48 (1.25–1.74)	<0.0001	Q5	>358	1.28 (1.04–1.58)	0.0181
[c]QT_{oa} (ms)	Q5	>268	1.46 (1.24–1.72)	<0.0001	Q5	>273	1.30 (1.06–1.59)	0.0116
[d]$\Theta(R\|STT)$	Q5	>79	1.52 (1.29–1.78)	<0.0001	Q5	>89	1.86 (1.54–2.25)	<0.0001
[e]$\Theta(T_p\|T_{ref})$	Q5	>25	1.51 (1.28–1.78)	<0.0001	Q5	>36	2.10 (1.74–2.54)	<0.0001
[f]$\Theta(T_{init}\|T_{term})$	Q5	>21	1.44 (1.22–1.70)	<0.0001	Q5	>25	1.70 (1.40–2.03)	<0.0001
[g]T_oV/TpV	Q5	>0.36	1.93 (1.42–2.63)	<0.0001	Q5	>0.41	1.87 (1.47–2.38)	<0.0001
[h]STJ aVR (μV)	Q5	>–5	1.37 (1.16–1.61)	0.0002	Q5	>4	1.64 (1.34–1.99)	<0.0001
[h]STJ V1 (μV)	Q5	>14	1.41 (1.19–1.67)	<0.0001	Q5	>19	1.51 (1.24–1.84)	<0.0001
[h]STJ V6 (μV)	Q1	<0	1.15 (0.97–1.37)	0.0979	Q1	<–10	2.01 (1.66–2.42)	<0.0001
Tampl. aVR (μV)	Q5	>–166	1.49 (1.26–1.75)	<0.0001	Q5	>–122	1.96 (1.62–2.37)	<0.0001
Tampl. aVL (μV)	Q1	<19	1.45 (1.23–1.71)	<0.0001	Q1	<–19	1.58 (1.30–1.91)	<0.0001

Tampl. V1 (μV)	Q5	>83	1.29 (1.09–1.52)	0.0033	Q5	>102	1.60 (1.32–1.95)	<0.0001
Tampl. V6 (μV)	Q1	<41	1.60 (1.36–1.88)	<0.0001	Q1	<87	1.89 (1.56–2.29)	<0.0001
[i]RT_{epi} (ms)	Q5	>350	1.43 (1.21–1.70)	<0.0001	–	–	–	–
[i]RT_{endo} (ms)	Q5	>383	1.36 (1.15–1.61)	0.0003	–	–	–	–
QRS dur. (ms)	–	–	–	–	Q5	>94	1.39 (1.13–1.70)	0.0022
[j]RNDPV	–	–	–	–	Q5	>57	1.41 (1.14–1.73)	0.0013
[h]STJV (μV)	–	–	–	–	Q5	>50	1.61 (1.31–1.96)	<0.0001
[h]STJaVL (μV)	–	–	–	–	Q1	<–10	1.33 (1.09–1.61)	<0.0001

From Rautaharju et al. [8]

CHD coronary heart disease, *CVD* cardiovascular disease, *HR* hazard ratio, *CI* 95 % confidence interval

[a]Test group threshold for the quintile (Q) listed with the remaining four quintiles as the reference group

[b]The risk for CHD death from a single ECG variable model multivariable-adjusted for study arm, age, race, smoke status, diabetes, hypertension, family history of CHD/stroke, body mass index and total cholesterol; ECG variables with low correlations were entered simultaneously into the multiple ECG variable model adjusting each of them to the other ECG variables and subsequently multivariable-adjusted to the same set of demographic/clinical variables as the single ECG variable model

[c]QT_{ea}, QT_{pa} and QT_{oa} = rate adjusted QTend (QT_e), QTpeak (QT_p) and QTonset (QT_o) whereby $QT_{ea} = QT_e + 184*(1\text{-}RR)$, $QT_{pa} = QT_p + 135*(1\text{-}RR)$ and $QT_{oa} = QT_o + 113*(1\text{-}RR)$

[d]$\Theta(R|STT)$ = spatial angle between mean QRS and ST-T vectors

[e]$\Theta(T_p|T_{ref})$ = spatial angle between T_p vector and the T reference (T_{ref}) vector

[f]$\Theta(T_{init}|T_{term})$ = spatial angle between the initial T vectors from quintiles 1 to 3 and terminal T vectors from quintiles 4 to 5

[g]T_oV/TpV = ratio of ToV and TpV vector magnitudes

[h]STJ refers to ST onset (J-point) amplitudes in the leads listed

[i]RT_{epi} and RT_{endo} are ECG estimates of epicardial and endocardial repolarization times, respectively (See Methods)

[j]RNDPV = QRS non-dipolar voltage from singular value decomposition (square root of pooled variance of components

4.3.2 *Independent Predictors of Coronary Heart Disease Death in Women*

Two alternative sets with pair-wise correlations <0.4 in each set were identified (Table 4.3): Set 1, Θ(Tp|Tref), the spatial angle between Tpeak (T_p) and normal T reference (T_{ref}) vectors, Θ(Tinit|Tterm), the spatial angle between the initial and terminal T vectors, and STJ depression in V6; and Set 2, TaVR and TV1 amplitudes, heart rate and QRS duration. $\Theta(T_{p|}T_{ref})$ >42° from Set 2 variables and TaVR amplitude less negative than −100 μV from Set 2 were the strongest independent predictors in women with and without CVD with an over twofold increased risk for both.

Table 4.3 Hazard ratios with 95 % confidence intervals for two sets of independent predictors of CHD death with common test group cut-off points at 95th or 5th percentiles in CVD-free women by CVD status at baseline

Variable (cutpoint)	CVD-free women		Women with CVD	
	Model 1[a]	Model 2[a]	Model 1[a]	Model 2[a]
Set 1				
[b]$\Theta(T_{p\|}T_{ref})$ (>42°)	2.13 (1.72–2.64)	1.73 (1.36–2.21)	2.03 (1.68–2.46)	1.49 (1.20–1.87)
[c]$\Theta(T_{init}\|T_{term})$ (>30°)	1.49 (1.19–1.86)	1.40 (1.08–1.80)	1.42 (1.14–1.75)	1.40 (1.11–1.78)
STJampl.V6 (<–25 μV)	1.30 (1.00–1.67)	1.07 (0.79–1.44)	1.62 (1.32–1.98)	1.75 (1.39–2.20)
Heart rate (>84/min)	1.87 (1.47–2.37)	1.54 (1.18–2.02)	1.10 (0.80–1.51)	0.95 (0.67–1.35)
[d]QT_{pa} (≥360 ms)	1.49 (1.27–1.76)	1.37 (1.13–1.65)	1.29 (1.07–1.56)	1.23 (0.99–1.52)
[e]*Set 2*				
Tampl. aVR (>–100)	2.27 (1.86–2.77)	1.81 (1.44–2.27)	2.09 (1.75–2.49)	1.71 (1.40–2.10)
Tampl. V1 (>175 μV)	1.56 (1.25–1.96)	1.41 (1.09–1.83)	1.85 (1.49–2.29)	1.54 (1.21–1.96)
Heart rate >84/min	2.25 (1.80–2.83)	1.78 (1.38–2.30)	1.30 (0.96–1.76)	1.14 (0.82–1.59)
QRS duration (≥100 ms)	1.64 (1.31–2.05)	1.35 (1.04–1.75)	1.45 (1.17–2.49)	1.45 (1.14–1.84)

From Rautaharju et al. [9]

CHD coronary heart disease, *CVD* cardiovascular disease, *HR* hazard ratio, *CI* confidence interval

[a]A set of ECG variables with low correlations (r<0.4) were entered simultaneously into the risk model and each was adjusted for the other ECG variables with no further adjustment (Model 1) and with additional adjustment for demographic and clinical factors (Model 2)

[b]$\Theta(T_p|T_{ref})$ = spatial angle between T peak (Tp) and T reference (Tref) vectors signifying deviation of repolarization direction in normal repolarization

[c]$\Theta(T_{init}|T_{term})$ = spatial angle between the mean initial and terminal T vectors from quintiles 1 to 3 and 4 to 5, respectively

[d]QTpa = rate-adjusted QTpeak interval

[e]$\Theta(T_{p|}T_{ref})$, $\Theta(T_{init}|T_{term})$ and STJ V6 were replaced in Set 2 by T amplitudes in aVR and V1

In CVD-free women also heart rate >84 had an over twofold increased risk among Set 2 variables. From clinical perspective an important observation was that TaVR was as strong predictors for the risk of CHD death as the computationally more complex variable Θ(Tp|Tref). TaVR amplitude may be a good choice for identification of women with high risk for CHD death for more diagnostic testing and possibly for more intensive intervention on CHD risk factors. In evaluation of potential adverse effects of cardioactive drugs other ECG predictors from the repolarization model may also warrant consideration particularly on Θ(Tp|Tref).

4.4 Sex Differences in Predictors for Coronary Heart Disease Death in Middle-Aged Men and Women

4.4.1 Single ECG Variable Predictors for Coronary Heart Disease Death

Data on CHD risk predictors in CVD-free men and women from a report from the Arteriosclerosis Research in Communities (ARIC) study were used to compare the predictors for CHD death in middle-aged men and women (Table 4.4). The table lists significant predictors of CHD death in men and women from single ECG variable risk models after multivariable adjustment for demographic/clinical factors. ECG procedures and the variables evaluated in ARIC and WHI studies were closely identical. In Table 4.4 gender-specific cutoff values for the test group were applied at 80th percent limit as indicated. Five of the ECG variables were significant predictors for CHD death in both sex groups. From these five, the strongest predictor was Θ(Rm|Tm), the spatial angle between the mean QRS and T vectors, with 2.32-fold increased risk in women and 3.85-fold increased risk in men. The other common significant predictors were the T wave deviation angles Θ(Tp|Tref) and Θ(Tinit|Tterm), TaVR amplitude and the spatial vector magnitude at ST onset, the J-point. All of these five ECG variables were strong predictors both in women and men although the HRs were higher in men than in women.

Additional three significant predictors in men only were prolonged QTea, the rate-adjusted QTend, prolonged RTepi, the epicardial repolarization time and increased ToV. Prolonged RTepi reflects delayed end of repolarization of the myocyte layers of the left ventricular lateral wall where repolarization normally starts earliest. ToV is the magnitude of the spatial vector magnitude curve at the onset of the T wave. Its increased value signifies reduction of the curvature of the ST vector magnitude curve between STo and Tp, thought to reflect triangularization of Phase 3 of the action potentials of the left ventricular lateral wall myocytes.

Overall, although the HRs for CHD death when evaluated as single variables were somewhat stronger in men than in women, the risk levels for ECG predictors in women are by no means negligible. This assertion becomes evident in the following section from evaluation of independent ECG predictors in women and men.

Table 4.4 Significant predictors of CHD death in men and women from single ECG variable risk models after multivariable adjustment for demographic/clinical factors

	Women		Men	
Variable (cutpoints)[a]	HR	95 % CI	HR	95 % CI
[b]Θ(Rm|Tm) (>53°/71°)	2.32	(1.59–3.39)	1.46	(1.09–1.95)
[c]Θ(Tp|Tref) (31°/31°)	1.61	(1.09–2.36)	1.85	(1.39–2.46)
[d]Θ(Tinit|Tterm) (>22°/>24°)	1.81	(1.23–2.66)	1.58	(1.18–2.11)
TaVR amplitude (>–136 μV/>–146 μV)	1.54	(1.05–2.25)	1.66	(1.25–2.22)
[e]QTea (>437 ms/>426 ms)	1.25	(0.85–1.85)	1.49	(1.11–2.00)
[f]RTepi (>347 ms/>329 ms)	1.33	(0.90–1.98)	1.40	(1.09–1.97)

HR was evaluated for increased values of the ECG parameters (quintile 5) as the test group, with quintiles 1–4 as the reference group

Single ECG variables multivariable-adjusted for age, race, education level, smoking status, alcohol status, asthma, cancer, diabetes, hypertension, family history of CHD and stroke, body mass index, systolic and diastolic blood pressure, high-density lipoprotein, low-density lipoprotein, triglycerides, white blood count, glucose, creatinine, and uric acid

HRs were evaluated for quintile 5 as the test group, with the remaining four quintiles as the reference group

CHD coronary heart disease, *HR* hazard ratio, *CI* confidence interval

[a]Cutpoints (in brackets) for test groups refer to the 80th percentile limits in women and men, respectively

[b]Θ(Rm|Tm) = spatial angle between mean QRS and T vectors

[c]Θ(Tp|Tref) = spatial angle between Tp vector and the T reference (Tref) vector

[d]Θ(Tinit|Tterm), spatial angle between the initial T vectors from quintiles 1–3 and the terminal T vectors from quintiles 4–5

[e]QTea = rate-adjusted QTe where QTea = QTe+127*(1-RR) for men and QTea = QTe+136*(1-RR) for women

[f]RTepi = epicardial repolarization time

Sex differences in SCD predictors are highlighted in Fig. 4.2 for those predictors which were significant either in women or men.

4.5 Independent Predictors of the Risk for Coronary Heart Disease Death in Women Free-from Cardiovascular Disease Compared to Men

Independent predictors for CHD were obtained by entering the predictors which were significant in univariate analysis simultaneously into the Cox regression model and adjusting each variable to other significant predictors (Table 4.5). Θ(Rm|Tm, the spatial angle between the mean QRS and T vectors was an independent predictor of CHD with a 2.04-fold increased risk in women and 1.62-fold increased risk in men. The risk for Θ(Tp|Tref) was increased 1.70-fold in women and 1.50-fold in men. TV1 amplitude in women and TaVR amplitude in men had an over twofold increased risk. QTea was not a significant predictor in women but it was an independent predictor for CHD death in men, with an over twofold increased risk.

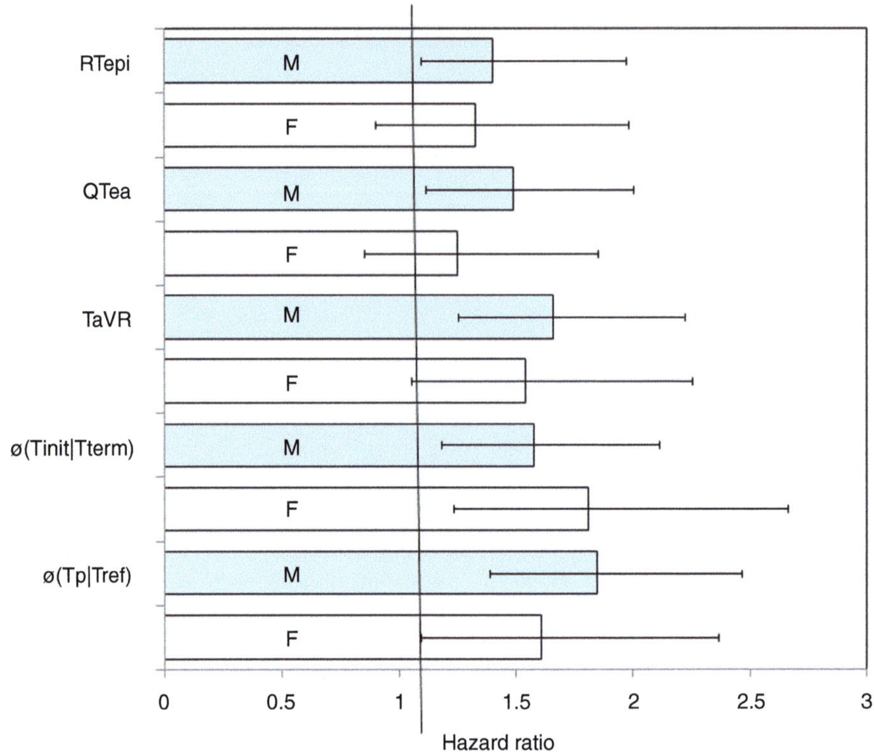

Fig. 4.2 Sex differences in sudden cardiac death predictors which were significant either in women or men

Table 4.5 Independent predictors of CHD death in CVD-free women and men

Women		Men	
Predictors	HR (95 % CI)	Predictors	HR (95 % CI)
[a]Θ(Rm|Tm) ≥53°	2.04*** (1.36, 3.07)	[a]Θ(Rm|Tm) ≥53°	1.40* (1.03–1.92)
[b]Θ(Tp|Tref) >31°	1.70* (1.11, 2.62)	[b]$\Theta(T_p\|T_{ref})$ >33°	1.40 (0.98–1.98)
TV1 ampl. ≥100 μV	2.03*** (1.40, 2.96)	TaVR ≥150 μV	1.54* (1.10–2.14)
		QTea >425 ms	1.48* (1.09–2.02)

Independent predictors were obtained by entering the predictors which were significant in univariate analysis simultaneously into the Cox regression model and adjusting each variable to other significant predictors. Hazard ratios were evaluated for quintile 5 with quintiles 1–4 as the referent except with quintiles 2–5 as the referent and quintile 1 as the test group for QT_{oa}, T_oV and TaVL
Modified from Table 6, Rautaharju et al. [9]

CHD coronary heart disease, *CVD* cardiovascular disease, *HR* hazard ratio, *CI* confidence interval
*Denotes $p<0.05$, ** $p<0.01$, ***$p<0.001$, otherwise non-significant for hazard ratios
[a]Θ(Rm|Tm) = spatial angle between mean QRS and T vectors
[b]$\Theta(T_p|T_{ref})$ = spatial angle between T_p vector and unit T_{ref} vector with x,y,z components (0.686, 0.528,–0.501) defining the normal direction of repolarization

References

1. Keys A, Aravanis C, Blackburn H, van Buchem FSP, Buzina R, Djordjevic BS, Fidanza F, Karvonen M, Menotti A, Puddu V, Taylor H. Probability of meddle-aged men developing coronary heart disease in five years. Circulation. 1972;45:815–26.
2. Multiple Risk Factor Intervention Trial Group. The Multiple Risk Factor Intervention Trial (MRFIT). A national study of primary prevention of coronary heart disease. J Am Med Assoc. 1976;235:825–7.
3. The Women's Health Initiative Study Group. Design paper. Design of the women's health initiative clinical trial and observational study. Control Clin Trials. 1998;19:61–109.
4. Mosca L, Barret-Connor E, Wenger NK. Sex/gender differences in cardiovascular disease prevention. What a difference a decade makes. Circulation. 2011;124:2145–54.
5. Ford ES, Capewell S. Coronary heart disease mortality among young adults in the U.S. from 1980 through 2002: concealed leveling of mortality rates. J Am Coll Cardiol. 2007;50:2128–32.
6. Rautaharju PM, Kooperberg C, Larson JC, LaCroix A. Electrocardiographic abnormalities that predict coronary heart disease events and mortality in postmenopausal women. The women's health initiative. Circulation. 2006;113:473–80.
7. Rautaharju PM, Zhang ZM. Linearly scaled, rate-invariant normal limits for QT interval. Eight decades of incorrect application of power functions. J Cardiovasc Electrophysiol. 2002;13:1211–8.
8. Rautaharju P, Zhang ZM, Vitolins M, Perez M, Allison M, Greenland P, Soliman E. Electrocardiographic repolarization-related variables as predictors of coronary heart disease death in the Women's Health Initiative (WHI) study. Am Heart Assoc. 2014 Jul 28;3(4). pii: e001005. doi: 10.1161/JAHA.114.001005.
9. Rautaharju PM, Zhan SM, Warren J, Gregg RE, Haisty Jr WK, Kurchanska-Newton AM, Rosamond WD, Soliman EZ. Electrocardiographic predictors of coronary heart disease and sudden cardiac deaths in men and women free from cardiovascular disease in the Atherosclerosis Risk in Communities study. J Am Heart Assoc. 2013;2(3):e000061. PubMed: PMID: 23723252.

Chapter 5
ECG Predictors of Atrial Fibrillation and Heart Failure

Synopsis The relatively high prevalence of atrial fibrillation (AF) and the associated impaired quality of life particularly in older women signifies the importance of this condition and its prevention. In age groups older than 75 years approximately 60 % of all AF patients are women. AF is associated with increased risk of CVD death and in some large population studies the risk has been found to be higher in women than in men.

The majority of older women and men with AF have a clinically manifest CVD or subclinical manifestations of CVD revealed by history and by a careful clinical evaluation. Lone AF is rare in elderly persons. Echocardiograhic and other imaging procedures will effectively identify subclinical CVD. Consideration of diagnostic procedures required for confirmation of clinical CVD and initiation of more effective therapeutic procedures seems warranted in patients with AF. AF treatment in women has been found more conservative than in men and intervention is delayed more commonly in women than in men although restoration of the sinus rhythm with electrical cardioversion has been found equally successful in women and men.

Abbreviations and Acronyms

AF	Atrial fibrillation
ARIC	Arteriosclerotic heart risk in communities study
CHS	Cardiovascular health study
CVD	Cardiovascular disease
HF	Heart failure
LBBB	Left bundle branch block
LVH	Left ventricular hypertrophy
MESA	Multi-ethnic study of atherosclerosis
MI	Myocardial infarction
MRI	Magnetic resonance imaging
TIA	Transient ischemic attack

P.M. Rautaharju, *The Female Electrocardiogram: Special Repolarization Features, Gender Differences, and the Risk of Adverse Cardiac Events*,
DOI 10.1007/978-3-319-15293-6_5

5.1 Introduction and Background

Atrial fibrillation (AF) and heart failure (HF) are evaluated here together because pathophysiological/hemodynamic factors in these two conditions interact when AF and HF coexist. A more comprehensive coverage of AF and other supraventricular dysrhythmias can be found in many other sources (including Rautaharju and Rautaharju [1]).

The evolution of hypertensive heart disease and development of left ventricular hypertrophy (LVH) play an important role in the mechanism for HF. These aspects are covered in Chap. 7. The importance of left bundle branch block (LBBB) as a predictor of HF is covered in Chap. 8. Although AF is not a short-terms causal factor for acute fatal events, identification of predictors of AF is still an important area of cardiac research. Preventing AF would have a more important impact on public health than attempts to prevent adverse cardiovascular (CVD) events after AF occurs. The relatively high prevalence of AF and the associated impaired quality of life particularly in older women signifies the importance of this condition and its prevention. From various supraventricular arrhythmias only atrial fibrillation will be considered here.

The quality of life of women with AF is more impaired than in men. In the Canadian Trial of Atrial Fibrillation the quality of life was evaluated at baseline, 3 and 6 months after antiarrhythmic drug treatment [2]. At the baseline the reported physical health and functional capacity in women after controlling for clinical and demographic factors was worse compared to those reported by men but there was no significant gender difference in reported mental health or general well-being. Women also had significantly more frequent and more severe cardiac symptoms than men. Physical health improved significantly from baseline to 3 months in women but not in men and conversely, mental health improved for men but not for women $p<0.001$ for all. Cardiac symptom frequency and severity improved over time for women and men. Gender difference in the reported quality of life is in part due to the tendency in women to somatize, i.e., to amplify bodily sensations but the gender difference in quality of life remained significant after controlling for somatization. Women with AF have a high risk of stroke, in women older than 75 years particularly embolic stroke [3]. AF treatment in women has been found more conservative with less rhythm control than in men and intervention is more commonly delayed in women [4] although restoration of sinus rhythm with electrical cardioversion has been found equally successful in women than in men [2].

AF is generally a manifestation of evolving subclinical CVD or has already clinically manifest CVD. Of the 141 women with AF in the 1994 report from CHS referred to above [5], 54 % had a clinical CVD and another 40 % had subclinical CVD. Clinical CVD diagnosis included a history of myocardial infarction (MI), silent ECG-MI, history of angina pectoris, stroke, transient ischemic attack (TIA), congestive heart failure, rheumatic heart disease, intermittent claudication, history of coronary artery bypass graft operation, percutaneous coronary artery angioplasty, carotid endarterectomy, and angioplasty or bypass surgery of arteries in leg. Three subsets of conditions defined subclinical CVD: (1) subclinical atrial/valvular disease (abnormal mitral or aortic valve function or abnormal left atrial dimension on M-mode echocardiogram); (2) subclinical ventricular disease (abnormal left ventricular wall motion of ejection fraction on echocardiogram or abnormal left ventricular mass (≥192.3 g in women and 256.3 g in men; 80th percentile by gender); and (3) subclinical atherosclerotic disease (ultrasound-defined carotid stenosis (≥25 % on either side), ankle-arm index <0.9, or gender-specific common or internal carotid artery mean intimal-medial thickness above 8th percentile.

5.2 Correlates of Atrial Fibrillation

Significant correlates of AF were evaluated in CHS by Furberg et al. [5]. Logistic regression was used to estimate odds ratios for the association between AF and various risk factors, clinical and subclinical diseases. In this sequential selection procedure factors with significant univariate correlation with AF the factors with significant correlation with AF in the final multivariate model were called 'correlators'. The following significant correlators were identified: (a) from clinical factors congestive heart failure and rheumatic heart disease; (b) from subclinical factors mitral stenosis, left atrial dimension and aortic regurgitation; and (c), from CVD risk factors, only treated hypertension remained a significant AF correlator. This sequential stepwise selection scheme excluded the following factors which were significantly associated with AF as single factors: (a) from clinical factors myocardial infarction and angina; (b) from subclinical factors abnormal ejection fraction, abnormal wall motion and left ventricular mass; and (c) from HF risk factors diabetes and serum glucose.

The results from this CHS report demonstrated that most elderly persons with AF have clinically confirmed CVD and that AF patients without clinically manifest CVD had subclinical CVD. Thus, lone AF is rare in elderly persons. A careful history and physical examination are the cornerstones in identification of clinical CVD. Echocardiograhic and other imaging procedures will effectively identify subclinical CVD. Consideration of these diagnostic procedures seems warranted in patients with AF. AF by self-report may be less accurate although careful consideration of prescribed medication use will increase the confidence in AF by self-report. Also, consideration should be given to the fact that AF is often transient as shown by ambulatory 24-h recordings [6].

In a 1997 report from the ARIC population [7] incident AF was strongly associated with age and its prevalence was lower in women than in men (10.1 and 21.6 per 1,000 person-years in women 65–74 and 75–84 years, respectively, and in men 17.6 and 42.7, respectively). Among other factors diuretic use, valvular heart disease and CHD, systolic blood pressure, glucose and left atrial size were associated with increased risk of AF in stepwise models. In their conclusions the authors emphasized the importance of left atrial size as an important risk factor for incident AF and potential importance of blood pressure control and glucose in preventing the development of AF.

5.3 Predictors and Precipitating Factors for Atrial Fibrillation: Integration of Concepts

Pathophysiological and functional interactions involved in the relationships between AF and HF are complex and there are conceptual problems in evaluation and interpreting clinical and ECG correlates and predictors of AF and HF. The block diagram in Fig. 5.1 shows the pathways of evolution from a CVD-free status to a condition where HF and AF are combined forming the vicious circle as noted above. Concerning AF and HF, the question remains which condition is the cause and which is the consequence. Impaired hemodynamics in AF includes high heart rate, reduced LV filling time and cardiac output. Loss of effective atrial contraction is detrimental particularly in patients with diastolic HF. In patients with HF and normal sinus rhythm the onset of new AF worsens cardiac function, peak oxygen consumption and mitral and aortic regurgitation [8]. Age, hypertension and diabetes as well as conditions precipitating structural myocardial abnormalities are common risk factors for AF and HF and the associated electrophysiological and neurohormonal alterations create a vicious circle whereby AF and HF further aggravate each other [9].

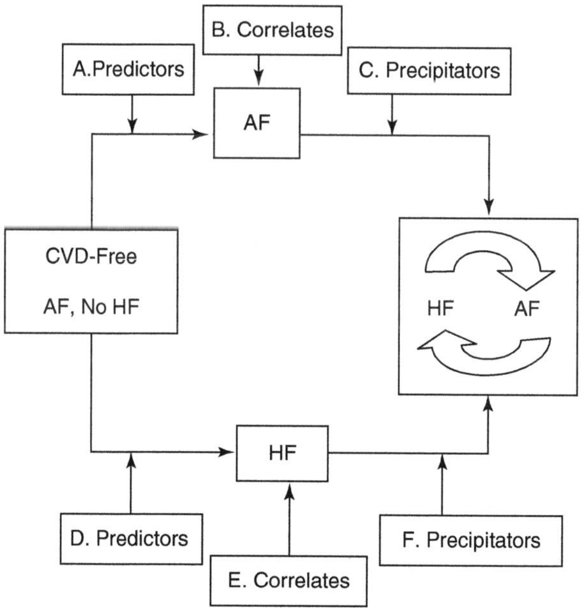

Fig. 5.1 A block diagram of the pathways of evolution from CVD-free status to atrial fibrillation (*AF*) and heart failure (*HF*) showing target locations for the search of ECG predictors of new-onset AF (*A*), the correlates of prevalent AF (*B*), precipitating ECG factors for HF in AF (*C*), predictors of new-onset HF (*D*), correlates of prevalent HF (*E*) and precipitating ECG factors for AF in HF (*F*)

Breaking this vicious circle is clinically a difficult patient management problem. From the perspective of public health preventing AF and HF as early on along the pathways of evolution is a desirable goal. For this reason identification of predictors of AF and HF before they occur is a high priority. Identification of possible ECG predictors of AF and HF is directly relevant for the objectives of this monograph.

5.4 ECG Predictors of Atrial Fibrillation and Heart Failure

ECG predictors of AF and HF from the ARIC studies are listed in Table 5.1. The first study by Soliman et al. [10] evaluated the risk for ECG predictors of AF in ARIC participants excluding those with AF at baseline. The primary objective of the study was to evaluate black and white differences in AF predictors and racial differences in AF risk and the risk of ischemic stroke. The study does not fully meet the requirements for AF predictors in CVD-free participants (box A in Fig. 5.1) although in incident AF analysis the risk for incident AF was evaluate by risk models after adjustment for age, sex, race and clinical factors. There were three main predictors of incident AF listed in Table 5.1. The maximum P wave duration in all ECG leads was associated with an over fourfold increased risk. In comparison the risk for P duration in lead II, a more commonly used ECG criterion for right atrial enlargement (RAE) was comparable, 3.9-fold increase. The risk for AF for P′APD, the P-prime amplitude-duration product was increased 90 %. This product, commonly labeled as PV1 terminal force, is used as a criterion for left atrial enlargement. It is of interest that P′ADP was also a predictor of ischemic stroke in the study of Soliman et al.

The second ARIC study [11] in Table 5.1 fits the requirements for predictors of incident HF (box E in Fig. 5.1) for estimating significant independent ECG predictors of HF. Increased QRS nondipolar voltage and two angular variables, ϴ(Rm|Tm) and ϴ(Tp|Tref) in women were independent predictors of HF, with an approximately 60 % increased risk for all. Prolonged RTepi, left ventricular epicardial repolarization time and prolonged TpTe interval in men were independent predictors of incident HF, with 62 % increased risk for RTepi and 27 % increased risk for TpTe interval. The latter variable reflects global dispersion of the end of repolarization. Two other ECG variables in men were also significant independent predictors: increased ϴ(Tp|Tref) and T wave complexity, with an approximately 30 % increased risk for both.

5.5 Heart Rate and Heart Failure: An Important Association Commonly Overlooked

Fatal and nonfatal outcomes associated with increased heart rate was evaluated in the Framingham study during two Decades of follow-up in 4,048 participants (mean age 55 years, 56 % women) [12]. New onset incident CVD was observed in 708

Table 5.1 Electrocardiographic predictors of incident atrial fibrillation and heart failure in the Atherosclerosis Risk in Communities (ARIC) study

	Predictor	Hazart ratio (95 % CI)	Comments
Endpoint: incident AF/study: Soliman et al. [10]/population: white and black ARIC participants (n = 15,429, mean follow-up 7 years)	*Women and men*		
	[a]P′ADPV1 (μV.s)	1.90 (1.02–3.66)	HR for >95 percentile vs. ≤95th percentile; adjusted for age, sex, race and clinical factors
	[b]MaxPdur (ms)	4.07 (2.55–6.51)	
	Pdur II (ms)	3.90 (2.42–6.27)	Compared to whites odds ratio for age- and sex-adjusted PdurII >95 % limit 2.6 (2.3–3.1) in blacks
Endpoint: incident HF/study: Rautaharju et al. [11]/population: ARIC participants, CVD-free subgroup (n = 13,428, follow-up 14 years)/incident HF	*Women*		
	[c]RNDPV >54 μV	1.46 (1.24–0.73)	HR for quintile 5 vs. the rest
	[d]Θ(Rm|Tm) >64°	1.54 (1.29–1.85)	
	[e]Θ(Tp|Tref) >28°	1.46 (1.21–1.76)	
	Men		
	[f]RTepi >329 ms	1.62 (1.34–1.97)	
	[g]TpTe >110 ms	1.27 (1.06–1.54)	
	Θ(Tp|Tref) >28°	1.31 (1.07–1.61)	
	[h]T wave complexity	1.32 (1.10–1.58)	

[a]P′ADPV1 = P′ wave amplitude-duration product in V1 (commonly labeled as P terminal force)
[b]MaxPdur = maximum P wave duration in 12-leads (excluding aVR)
[c]RNDPV = QRS nondipolar voltage from singular value decomposition
[d]Θ(Rm|Tm) = spatial angle between the mean QRS and T vectors
[e]Θ(Tp|Tref) = spatial angle between Tp and Tref vectors, indicating T wave deviation angle of Tp vector from Tp in normal repolarization with unit vector xyz components (0.66, 0.48, –0.67)
[f]RTepi = epicardial repolarization time from the repolarization model
[g]TpTe = TpTe interval reflecting global dispersion of the end of repolarization
[h]T wave complexity = ratio of the second and first principal components of T wave reflecting the roundness of T vector loop

participants, 303 of them HF. In Cox risk models with multivariable adjustment for clinical risk factors and physical activity participants with higher heart rate had an excess risk of CVD events largely due to incident HF. Participants in the highest quartile of heart rate (>69/min for men and >74/min for women) had a twofold increased risk for HF.

There was no significant effect modification by sex implying that the risk for HF was equally strong for women and men. The authors note that heart rate from a single examination was as strong predictor of incident CVD as an average heart rate over an 8 year period.

Heart rate may directly affect CVD risk for instance through its association with progression of atherosclerosis [13]. Ingwall and Weiss in their review noted that the total creatine pool is decreased in human hearts in HF and the magnitude of the decrease is related to HF severity [14].

The association between heart rate, left ventricular (LV) dysfunction and HF was evaluated in the Multiethnic Study of Atherosclerosis (MESA) by Opdahl et al. [15]. Incident HF was observed during the median follow-up of 7 years in 176 of 5,000 study participant who were examined by cardiac magnetic resonance imaging (MRI). LV dysfunction was measured by development of regional and global LV circumferential strain. There was a 40 % greater adjusted risk for incident HF for 10 bpm increase in resting heart rate. Resting heart rate was positively associated with HF and deteriorating LV circumferential strain and the association remained significant even when CHD events were excluded from the model.

5.6 Dyssynchrony of Ventricular Excitation and Contraction as Predictor of Sudden Cardiac Death

The importance of HF is emphasized by the fact that HF afflicts nearly six million Americans, resulting in one million emergency department visits and over one million annual hospital discharges [16]. Dyssynchrony or ventricular contraction has become an important consideration in resynchronization therapy of HF patients. The need for more effective diagnostic procedures including nuclear cardiology in patients with acute HF [17] and the choice of more effective therapeutic procedures has been clinically recognized [16]. In symptomatic patients with acute HF and reduced EF, left ventricular dyssynchrony is a predictor of sudden cardiac death.

References

1. Rautaharju P, Rautaharju F. Investigative electrocardiography in epidemiological studies and clinical trials. London: Springer; 2007. p. 1–289.
2. Paquette M, Roy D, Talajic M, Newman D, Couturier A, Yang C, Dorian P. Role of gender and personality on quality-of-life impairment in intermittent atrial fibrillation. Am J Cardiol. 2000;86:764–8.

3. Hart RG, Pearce LA, McBride R, Rothbart RM, Asinger RW. Factors associated with ischemic stroke during aspirin therapy in atrial fibrillation: analysis of 2012 participants in the SPAF I-III clinical trials. The Stroke Prevention in Atrial Fibrillation (SPAF) Investigators. Stroke. 1999;30:1223–9.
4. Dagres N, Nieuwlaat R, Vardas PE, Andresen D, Lévy S, Cobbe S, Kremastinos DT, Breithardt G, Cokkinos DV, Crijns HJ. Gender-related differences in presentation, treatment, and outcome of patients with atrial fibrillation in Europe: a report from the Euro Heart Survey on Atrial Fibrillation. J Am Coll Cardiol. 2007;49:572–7.
5. Furberg CD, Psaty BM, Manolio TA, Gardin JM, Smith VE, Rautaharju PM. Prevalence of atrial fibrillation in elderly subjects. The Cardiovascular Health Study. Am J Cardiol. 1994; 74:236–41.
6. Rautaharju PM, Manolio TA, Furberg CD, Siscovick D, Newman AB, Borhani NO, Gardin JM. Ischemic episodes in 24-hour ambulatory electrocardiograms of elderly persons: the Cardiovascular Health Study. Int J Cardiol. 1995;51:165–75.
7. Psaty BM, Manolio TA, Kuller LH, Cushman M, Fried LP, White R, Furberg CD, Rautaharju PM. The incidence of atrial fibrillation and risk factors for atrial fibrillation in older adults. Circulation. 1997;96:2455–61.
8. Pozzoli M, Cioffi G, Traversi E, Pinna GD, Cobelli F, Tavazzi L. Predictors of primary atrial fibrillation and concomitant clinical and hemodynamic changes in patients with chronic heart failure: a prospective study in 344 patients with baseline sinus rhythm. J Am Coll Cardiol. 1998;32:197–204.
9. Anter E, Jessup M, Callans DJ. Atrial fibrillation and heart failure. Treatment considerations for a dual epidemic. Circulation. 2009;119:2516–25.
10. Soliman EZ, Prineas RJ, Case LD, Zhang ZM, David C, Goff Jr DC. Ethnic distribution of ECG predictors of atrial fibrillation and its impact on understanding the ethnic distribution of ischemic stroke in the Atherosclerosis Risk in Communities (ARIC) study. Stroke. 2009;40: 1204–11.
11. Rautaharju PM, Zhang ZM, Haisty Jr EK, Prineas RJ, Kurchanska-Newton AM, Rosamond WD, Soliman EZ. Electrocardiographic predictors of incident heart failure in men and women free from manifest cardiovascular disease from the Atherosclerosis Risk in Communities [ARIC] study). Am J Cardiol. 2013;112:843–9.
12. Ho JE, Larson MG, Ghorbani A, Cheng D, Coglianese EE, Vasan RS, Wang TJ. Long-term cardiovascular risks associated with an elevated heart rate: the Framingham Heart Study. J Am Heart Assoc. 2014;3:e000668. doi:10.1161/JAHA.113.000668.
13. Giannoglou GD, Chatzizisis YS, Zamboulis C, Parcharidis GE, Mikhailidis DP, Louridas GE. Elevated heart rate and atherosclerosis: an overview of the pathogenetic mechanisms. Int J Cardiol. 2008;126:302–12.
14. Ingwall JS, Weiss RG. Is the failing heart energy starved? On using chemical energy to support cardiac function. Circ Res. 2004;95:135–45.
15. Opdahl A, Venkatesh BA, Fernandes VRS, Wu CO, Nasir K, Choi E-Y, Almeida ALC, Rosen B, Carvalho B, Edvardsen T, Bluemke DA, Lima JAC. Resting heart rate as predictor for left ventricular dysfunction and heart failure in MESA (Multi-Ethnic Study of Atherosclerosis). J Am Coll Cardiol. 2014;63:1182–9.
16. Collins S, Storrow AB, Albert NM, Butler J, Ezekowitz J, Felker GM, SAEM/HFSA Acute Heart Failure Working Group, et al. Early management of patients with acute heart failure: state of the art and future directions. A consensus document from the Society for Academic Emergency Medicine/Heart Failure Society of America Acute Heart Failure Working Group. J Card Fail. 2015;21:27–43.
17. Hage FG, Aggarwal H, Patel K, Chen J, Jacobson AF, Heo J, Ahmed A, Iskandrian AE. The relationship of left ventricular mechanical dyssynchrony and cardiac sympathetic denervation to potential sudden cardiac death events in systolic heart failure. J Nucl Cardiol. 2014;21:78–85.

Chapter 6
ECG Predictors of Sudden Cardiac Death

Synopsis Sudden cardiac death (SCD), also labeled as primary cardiac arrest (PCA) is generally defined as sudden death occurring within 1 h after the onset of symptoms when no other cause of death is evident. SCD is often the first manifestation of coronary heart disease (CHD). From various arrhythmias ventricular tachycardia and ventricular fibrillation play an important role as mechanisms of SCD. QT prolongation is thought to be a marker of increased risk of SCD.

In a case-control study among patients who experienced SCD (including about 45 % women) treated for hypertension but free from recognized heart disease, the risk for SCD was increased after adjustment for other risk factors for three continuous variables: and index for QT prolongation (QTI), an index for cardiac injury containing a variety of ventricular excitation and repolarization variables and an ECG index for left ventricular hypertrophy containing the Cornell voltage and body weight. These variables were stronger predictors when used as continuous variables as the same variables used as dichotomized variables.

In another case-control study (32 % women) among diabetic patients excluding prior physician-diagnosed heart disease the risk for PCA was increased 3.5-fold in the fourth versus first QTI quartile, corresponding rate-adjusted QT prolongation 7 % above the QTI in reference normal men and women.

In the large Rotterdam Heart Study in 4,878 women and 3,105 men 55 years old and older, the multivariable-adjusted for risk for SCD was increased 2.5-fold. Stratified by sex and adjusted for age, the SCD risk was increased 2.5-fold in women and 2.6-fold in men.

In the Atherosclerosis Research in Communities (ARIC) Study in 7,684 middle-aged women and 5,937 men free from CVD at baseline, the strongest predictor of SCD in women and men was Θ(Tp|Tref) with 2.59-fold increased risk of SCD in women and 2.22-fold increased risk in men. Θ(Tp|Tref) is a measure of deviant spatial direction of the regional repolarization sequence in the lateral wall of the left ventricle. TaVR amplitude was a significant predictor of SCD in women (2.59-fold increased risk) and in men (2.2-fold increased risk). The rate-adjusted QTe was a significant predictor in men only (1.94-fold increased risk). Overall, increased TaVR amplitude was the most uniform predictor of CHD death and SCD in men and in women. The presence of a positive, flat or less negative than −100 μV (−1 mm) TaVR amplitude in men and women with CVD calls for additional diagnostic evaluation and possibly stronger therapeutic measures for prevention of CHD death and SCD.

P.M. Rautaharju, *The Female Electrocardiogram: Special Repolarization Features, Gender Differences, and the Risk of Adverse Cardiac Events*,
DOI 10.1007/978-3-319-15293-6_6

Abbreviations and Acronyms

ARIC	Arteriosclerosis research in communities
CHD	Coronary heart disease
DBP	Diastolic blood pressure
HR	Hazard ratio
PAR	Population attributable risk
PCA	Primary cardiac arrest
QTcBz	QTe adjusted by Bazett's formula
QTe	QTend interval
QTea	Rate-adjusted QTe
QTI	QT prolongation index
QTp	QTpeak interval
QTpa	Rate-adjusted QTp
SBP	Systolic blood pressure
SCD	Sudden cardiac death
VF	Ventricular fibrillation
VT	Ventricular tachycardia
WHI	Women's health initiative
Θ(Tinit|Tterm)	Spatial angle between the initial and terminal T vectors
Θ(Tp|Tref)	Spatial angle between Tp vector and the mean Tp vector in normal reference group (Tref)

6.1 Introduction

SCD is generally defined as sudden death occurring within 1 h after the onset of symptoms when no other cause of death is evident. From various arrhythmias ventricular tachycardia and ventricular fibrillation (VF) play an important role as mechanisms of sudden cardiac death (SCD). Ventricular ectopic (VE) activity is generally prognostically less important than other ventricular arrhythmias although frequent VEs have in some reports been found to predict adverse events such as incident stroke [1]. Ventricular arrhythmias include frequent VEs ventricular tachycardias (VT, runs of three or more VEs) and ventricular fibrillation (VF). Only VT and VF will be considered here in the context of sudden cardiac death (SCD). Epidemiological aspects of VE were covered in reference [2].

6.2 Sudden Cardiac Death: Prevalence and Risk Factors

A variety of factors have been related to the risk of SCD, including even less obvious factors such as diet. For the latter factor the association with SCD was evaluated in a prospective study in 93,122 postmenopausal women from the Women's Health

Initiative (WHI) study [3]. The average follow-up was 10.5 years. A score was assigned according to how closely the reported diet resembled the Mediterranean diet. A higher Mediterranean diet score was associated with lower risk of SCD (HR: 0.64; 95 % CI: 0.43–0.94) after adjustment for age, total energy, race, income, smoking, and physical activity.

Another prospective study in 161,808 women from the WHI clinical trials and observational studies estimated the annual incidence rate of SCD and identified risk factors for SCD [4]. The participants were enrolled between 1993 and 1998, and followed until August 2009. Incident SCD was defined as death occurring within 1 h of symptom onset or within 1 h after the participant was last seen without symptoms and death that occurred in the absence of a potentially lethal non-coronary disease process. Adjudicated SCD occurred in 418 women. Of interest was the fact that nearly one-half of women who experienced sudden cardiac death had no previous diagnosis of coronary heart disease. The incidence rate of SCD was 2.4/10,000 women/year (95 % confidence interval: 2.2–2.7). The study identified 11 independent risk factors for SCD including 6 traditional risk factors for CHD (older age, tobacco use, diabetes, history of myocardial infarction, previous CHD, and hypertension). Besides these risk factors for CHD, the additional risk factors for sudden cardiac death in postmenopausal women included African-American race, higher pulse, higher waist-to-hip ratio, elevated white blood cell count, and heart failure. Overall, population-attributable fractions were greatest for hypertension, waist-to-hip ratio, and myocardial infarction. Population attributable risk (PAR) was defined as:

$$\mathrm{PAR} = \left[\mathrm{Prev} \times \left(\mathrm{RR} - 1\right) / \mathrm{Prev} \times \left(\mathrm{RR} - 1\right) + 1\right],$$

where Prev is the prevalence of the exposure, and relative risk RR is the relative risk taken as the hazard [5].

Ventricular fibrillation (VF) is considered as the main mechanism of sudden cardiac arrhythmic death, and QT prolongation is thought to be a marker of increased risk for this fatal outcome. The mechanism of primary cardiac arrest is generally VF which in a strict sense is not a cardiac arrest. However, a person even immediately after the onset of ventricular fibrillation is found pulseless because in VF the left ventricular filling time is so short that no pulse is felt. This is why the condition is called cardiac arrest.

6.3 ECG Predictors of Sudden Cardiac Death

Some studies have focused specifically on ECG predictors of arrhythmic SCD often labeled as primary cardiac arrest (PCA). Table 6.1 is a summary table of selected studies on ECG predictors of arrhythmic SCD. The source data for the first two of the studies in the table come from a large prepaid health plan, Group Health Cooperative of Puget Sound in Seattle and surrounding King County, Washington.

Table 6.1 A summary table for selected reports on ECG predictors of SCD

Study	Predictor variables/ test group criteria	Hazard ratio (95 % CI)	Adjustment
Siscovick et al. [6]	[a]QTI	1.8 (1.3–2.7)	[d]Clinical factors
Group Health Cooperative of Puget Sound, WA	[b]CIIS	1.7 (1.2–2.5)	
Treated hypertensive patients, free from recognized heart disease	[c]LVMI	1.4 (1.0–2.0)	
Case-control study; cases (n=131), controls (n=562)	(Quintile 5 vs. quintile 1 for each criterion)		
Women 46 % of controls, 44 % of cases			
Whitsel et al. [11]	[e]QTI	Primary cardiac arrest risk increased 3.5-fold	[e]Sampling design, age, and race
Group Health Cooperative of Puget Sound, WA			
Enrollees with physician-diagnosed diabetes or treated with oral hypoglycemics or insulin. Enrollees with prior physician-diagnosed heart disease were excluded. Cases (n=79), controls (n=214). Women 32 % of cases and controls	Definite QT prolongation (QTI >107 %) vs. mean normal QTI (100 %)		
Rotterdam Heart Study. Straus et al. [12]. Women (n=4,878) and men (n=3,105), 55 years old and older; 125 SCD events during an average follow-up 6.7 years	QTcBz women and men	2.5 (1.3–4.7)	Demographic/ clinical factors
	QTcBz women	2.5 (1.0–7.1)	Age
	QTcBz men	2.6 (1.1–5.8)	Age
Baseline prevalence: hypertension 33.6 %, diabetes 10.5 %, ECG-MI 6.3 %, HF3.2 %,	Women QTcBz >470 ms vs. < 450 ms		
Definite prolonged QTcBz: 8.5 %	Men QTcBz >450 ms vs. <430 ms		
ARIC Study, Rautaharju et al. [13]	[f]Θ(Tp|Tref) women	2.59 (1.39–4.82)	Single ECG variable risk models multivariable-adjusted for demographic/clinical factors;

Table 6.1 (continued)

Study	Predictor variables/ test group criteria	Hazard ratio (95 % CI)	Adjustment
CVD-free subgroup of 5,937 men and 7,684 women, 45–65 years old, predominantly white (70 %), approximately 30 % hypertensives, 10 % diabetics. Average follow-up 14 years	[f]Θ(Tp|Tref) men	2.22 (1.43–3.43)	HR evaluated for quintile 5 for each predictor variable as the test group, with quintiles 1–4 as the reference group[i]
	[g]Θ(Tinit|Tterm) women	1.47 (0.79–2.72)	
	[g]Θ(Tinit|Tterm) men	1.68 (1.07–2.62)	
	TaVR women	1.79 (0.97–3.29)	
	TaVR men	1.64 (1.04–2.58)	
	[h]QTea women	1.18 (0.63–2.23)	
	[h]QTea men	1.94 (1.25–3.01)	

[a]*QTI* QT prolongation index [5]
[b]*CIIS* cardiac infarction/injury score [6]
[c]*LVMI* left ventricular mass index [7]
[d]Clinical characteristics, including age, sex, current smoking, diabetes, treated diastolic blood pressure, resting heart rate (for LVHI and CIIS), and antihypertensive therapy
[e]Conditional logistic regression models adjusted for sampling design, age, and race
[f]Θ(Tp|Tref) = spatial angle between Tpeak vector and the reference T vector(Tref) for normal spatial sequence of repolarization
[g]Θ(Tinit|Tterm) = spatial angle between the initial and terminal T vectors from quintiles 1 to 3 and 4 to 5 of repolarization, respectively
[h]QTea = rate-adjusted QT interval from formulas QTea = QT−435*($RR^{0.33}$−1) for women and QTea = QT−416*($RR^{0.33}$−1) for men
[i]Group-specific cutpoints for women and men for each predictor

In the first study listed in Table 6.1, Siscovick et al. performed a case-control study among patients with SCD [6]. The cases (n = 131) had had primary cardiac arrest and the controls (n = 562) were a stratified random sample. Both groups had been treated for hypertension but were free from recognized heart disease. From cases 44 % were women and from controls 46 %. Three ECG measures on a continuous scale were evaluated: QT prolongation by QT Index (QTI) [7], the severity level of cardiac injury by Cardiac Infarction/Injury Score (CIIS) [8] and ECG-LVH by Left Ventricular Mass Index (LVMI) [9]. The risk for primary cardiac arrest was evaluated by comparing the 80th percentile with the 20th percentile of each score. After adjustment for other risk factors and binary ECG criteria for the abnormalities, the risk was increased 40 % for LVHI, 70 % for CIIS and 80 % for QTI. These findings suggest that in addition to QT, continuous ECG measures such as CIIS containing selected repolarization abnormalities are sensitive predictors of SCD, and that dichotomized criteria for LVH, old MI and QT may underestimate the prognostic value of these ECG abnormalities.

Although not listed in Table 6.1, in an earlier study Siscovick et al. addressed the question whether treatment of diastolic blood pressure (DBP) below 85 mmHg is associated with increased risk of primary cardiac arrest [10]. There were a smaller group of cases with primary cardiac arrest between 1977 and 1990 (n = 80). Control patients were a stratified random sample of hypertensive enrollees (n = 426). Logistic regression models after adjustment for pretreatment diastolic blood pressure, antihypertensive therapy, and other potential confounders and compared with a treated DBP of 85 mmHg, a treated DBP of 80 mmHg was associated with a small increase in relative risk (RR) (RR 1.2, 95 % CI 1.0–1.6). A 75 mmHg treated DBP was associated with a modest increase in risk (RR 1.6, CI 1.2–2.1), a 70 mmHg treated DBP was associated with more than a twofold increase in the risk of primary cardiac arrest (RR 2.3, CI 1.4–3.8). There was little evidence of effect modification by pretreatment diastolic blood pressure. The authors concluded that among hypertensive patients a treated diastolic blood pressure level below 85 mmHg is associated with cardiac hazards.

6.4 ECG Predictors of Sudden Cardiac Death in Patients with Diabetes

The second study listed in Table 6.1 addresses the question of primary cardiac arrest in diabetic patients. Pathophysiological mechanisms of QT prolongation and the failure of the automatic nervous system are thought to account at least in part for increased risk of SCD particularly in diabetes, often as a joint manifestation of diabetes and CHD. Primary cardiac arrest can occur as the first manifestation of CHD. Whitsel et al. evaluated the risk for primary cardiac arrest in patients with physician-diagnosed diabetes or who were treated with oral hypoglycemics or insulin [11]. Excluded were enrollees with prior physician-diagnosed heart disease. The proportion of women was 32 % of cases and controls. In conditional logistic regression models adjusted for sampling design, age, and race, the risk for primary cardiac arrest was increased 3.5-fold in the fourth versus first QTI quartile. The 80th percentile limit for QTI identifying the fourth quartile was 107 %, indicating rate-adjusted QT prolongation exceeding 7 % above the QTI in reference normal men and women.

The authors conclude that QT prolongation may be useful in risk stratifying populations of predominantly white, type 2 diabetic patients for primary cardiac arrest. The question about the generalizability of the findings to diabetic patients who are nonwhite and those with prior angina, myocardial infarction, and/or congestive heart failure remains open.

6.5 Gender Differences in Predictors of Sudden Cardiac Death in a Large General Population Group

Two studies in Table 6.1 compared gender differences in predictors of SCD. The first study in the urban population, the Rotterdam Heart Study found a strong association between SCD and prolonged QT by the Bazett's formula (QTcBz) in 4,878 women and 3,105 men 55 years old and older [12]. The participants were examined between 1993 and 1995. The follow-up performed until January

1, 2000 (average 6.7 years) and during this period 125 participants died of SCD. Definite QT prolongation was defined by QTcBz >470 ms in women and >450 ms in men.

Close to a third of the study group (33.6 %) were hypertensive (using antihypertensive medication or systolic blood pressure (SBP) ≥160 mmHg or DBP ≥100 mmHg) ranging from 31 % among those with normal QT, 39 % in the group with borderline QT prolongation to 45 % among those with definite QT prolongation. The prevalence of diabetes mellitus was 10.5 %, myocardial infarction 6.3 % and heart failure 3.2 %.

In the combined group of women and men the risk for SCD adjusted for demographic/clinical factors was increased 2.5-fold (HR 2.5, CI 1.3–4.7). Stratified by sex and adjusted for age, the SCD risk was increased 2.5-fold in women (HR 2.5, CI 1.0–7.1) and 2.6-fold in men (HR 2.6, CI 1.1–5.8).

The question arises whether prolonged QT is the causative mechanism for SCD or merely a marker of underlying silent CHD or some other heart disease. Other ECG variables are often correlated with QT prolongation and adjustment for them does not necessary remove collinearity problems influencing the observed associations. Moss, in an editorial accompanying the article raises also raises the question whether the presence of one or more ion-channel gene polymorphisms could cause minor alterations in ion-channel function that contribute to modest prolongation in cardiac repolarization and increase the probability for fatal arrhythmias [11]. However, the prevalence of such genetic aberrations of ionic channel function is probably too low to account for CVD at population level. Also, the reported risk levels in the Rotterdam Heart Study for prolonged QT were very strong in women and men.

6.6 Gender Differences in Sudden Cardiac Death Predictors in Women and Men Free-from Cardiovascular Disease

The last entry in Table 6.1 comparing gender differences in the ECG predictors of SCD comes from the Atherosclerosis Research in Communities (ARIC) Study in middle-aged women and men free from CVD ate baseline [13]. Listed are significant predictors of SCD death from single ECG variable risk models after multivariable adjustment for demographic/clinical factors (age, race, education level, smoking status, alcohol status, asthma, cancer, diabetes, hypertension, family history of CHD and stroke, body mass index, systolic and diastolic blood pressure, triglycerides, high-density lipoprotein, low-density lipoprotein, white blood count, glucose, creatinine, and uric acid). The strongest predictor in women and men was Θ(Tp|Tref) with 2.59-fold increased risk of SCD in women and 2.22-fold increased risk in men. Θ(Tp|Tref) is a measure of deviant spatial direction of the regional repolarization sequence in the lateral wall of the left ventricle. Θ(Tinit|Tterm), the second angular measure of deviant repolarization sequence was significantly increased in men (1.68-fold) but not in women. A widened Θ(Tinit|Tterm) reflects roundness of the T vector loop, at times labeled T wave complexity. TaVR

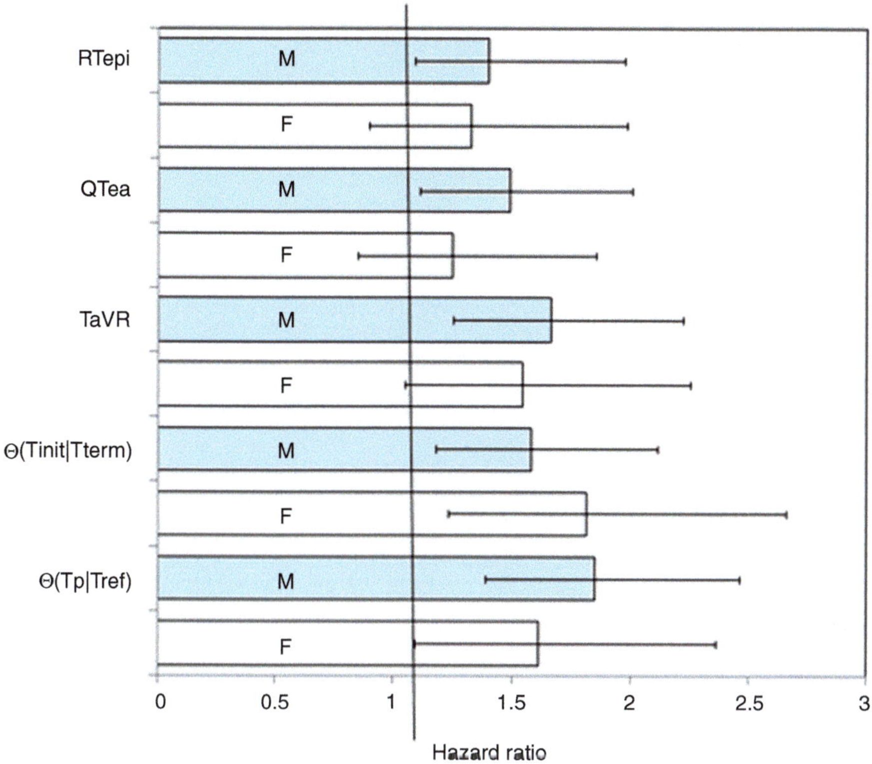

Fig. 6.1 Hazard ratios for ECG predictors of SCD in women (*white bars*) and men (*blue bars*) evaluated as single variables in risk models after multivariable adjustment for demographic/clinical factors. *Error bars* are for 96 % confidence limits. QTea is the rate-adjusted QTend interval, Θ(Tinit|Tterm) the spatial angle between the initial and terminal T vectors and Θ(Tp|Tref) is the spatial angle between Tpeak (*Tp*) vector and the mean Tp vector in normal reference group (*Tref*) (Modified from Table 6, Rautaharju et al. [13], with permission)

amplitude was a significant predictor of SCD in women (2.59-fold increased risk) and in men (2.2-fold increased risk). The rate-adjusted QTe was a significant predictor in men only (1.94-fold increased risk) (Fig. 6.1).

6.7 Independent Predictors of Sudden Cardiac Death in Women and Men Free-from Cardiovascular Disease

Independent predictors for SCD in the ARIC study cited in Table 6.1 were obtained by entering significant ECG variables in univariate analysis simultaneously into the Cox regression model and adjusting each variable to other significant predictors

Table 6.2 Independent predictors of CHD death and sudden cardiac death in CVD-free women and men

	CVD-free women		CVD-free men	
	[a]Independent predictors	Hazard ratio (95 % CI)	[a]Independent predictors	Hazard ratio (95 % CI)
CHD death	[b]Θ(Rm|Tm) ≥53°	2.04*** (1.36, 3.07)	[b]Θ(Rm|Tm) ≥53°	1.62* (1.03–255)
	[c]Θ(Tp|Tref) >31°	1.70* (1.11, 2.61)	[c]Θ(T_p|T_{ref}) >33°	1.50* (1.00–1.25)
	TV1 ampl. ≥100 μV	2.03*** (1.40, 2.96)	TaVR ≥150 μV	2.05* (1.20–3.49)
			QTea >425 ms	2.05 (1.20–3.49)
Sudden cardiac death	[c]Θ(Tp|Tref) >31°	3.55*** (1.85, 6.81)	[c]Θ(Tp|Tref) >33°	1.91* (1.14–3.20)
	[b]Θ(Rm|Tm) ≥53°	2.28* (1.17, 4.45)	[d]Θ(Tinit|Tterm) >24°	1.61* (11.01–2.56)
	TV1 ampl. ≥100 μV	2.26*** (1.20, 4.25)	[e]QTea >437 ms	1.98 (1.29–3.03)

Modified from Rautaharju et al. [13], with permission
CHD coronary heart disease, *CVD* cardiovascular disease
*Denotes $p<0.05$, ** $p<0.01$, ***$p<0.001$, otherwise non-significant for hazard ratios
[a]Independent predictors were obtained by entering the predictors which were significant in univariate analysis simultaneously into the Cox regression model and adjusting each variable to other significant predictors. Hazard ratios were evaluated for quintile 5 with quintiles 1–4 as the referent except with quintiles 2–5 as the referent and quintile 1 as the test group for QT_{oa}, T_oV and TaVL
[b]Θ(Rm|Tm) = spatial angle between mean QRS and T vectors
[c]Θ(T_p|T_{ref}) = spatial angle between T_p vector and unit T_{ref} vector with x,y,z components (0.686, 0.528, −0.501) defining the normal direction of repolarization
[d]Θ(Ti_{nit}|T_{term}) = spatial angle between initial and terminal T vectors
[e]QTea = rate-adjusted QTend interval

(Table 6.2). Hazard ratios listed are for quintile 5 as the test group using quintiles 1–4 as the reference. Sex-specific threshold values for cutoff points between the reference and test groups for each ECG predictor were as listed in the table. Θ(Tp|Tref) was the strongest independent predictor of SCD in CVD-free women with 3.55-fold increased risk. In CVD-free men, the risk for Θ(Tp|Tref) was increased 1.91-fold. It is noted that relatively small degree of deviancy from normal spatial direction of repolarization (>31° in women and >33° in men) is associated with increased risk for SCD.

The remaining independent predictors were different in women from those in men: Θ(Rm|Tm) and TV1 amplitude in women, and in men Θ(Tinit|Tterm) and QTea. A noteworthy observation is the 3.55-fold increased risk for SCD for Θ(Tp|Tref) in women. QTea was an independent predictor in men but not in women.

6.8 Sex Differences in Independent Predictors of CHD Death and SCD in Men and Women with CVD

In another ARIC study in participants with CVD (14), the selection from each pairs of highly correlated variables the more likely explanatory variables for SCD reduced the number of candidate variables for independent predictors of CHD death and SCD. This search was performed to avoid collinearity problems due to correlated variables ($r > 0.6$). Any remaining correlated variables in the final step of this search were placed in different sets of predictors. In the resulting primary set of independent predictors (Set 1) (Table 6.3) the strongest predictor was $\Theta(T_p|T_{ref})$ angle >54° with an over twofold increased risk for CHD death in women and a nearly fourfold increased risk in men. Two other independent predictors in women were ST J-point depression in V6 and QRS duration 102 ms or longer, with over twofold increased risk for both. From the alternative set (Set 2), TaVR and TV1 were strong independent predictors of CHD death in women.

From the primary set of independent predictors of SCD the risk in women was particularly pronounced for ToV/TpV ratio (7.76-fold increased risk) and also STJ depression in V6 was a strong predictor (4.48-fold increased risk). From the primary set of independent predictors of SCD in men Θ(Tp|Tref) was a strong and the only predictor (3.40-fold increased risk) and from Set 2 variables TaVR in men was a strong and the only independent predictor, with a threefold increased risk.

An important finding in Table 6.3 is that TaVR was the most consistent predictor overall, with approximately threefold increased risk in women and men for CHD death and for SCD.

Clinical Implications Overall, increased TaVR amplitude was as strong predictor of CHD death and SCD as computationally more complex angular variables in men and

Table 6.3 Hazard ratios (95 % confidence limits) for independent predictors of sudden cardiac death in ARIC study participants with cardiovascular disease at baseline by gender

	Threshold		Women		Men	
	Women	Men	HR	95 % CI	HR	95 % CI
TaVR (μV)	≥−68	≥−63	3.03*	(1.51–7.60)	3.00***	(1.71–5.24)
TV1 (μV)	≥102	≥110	3.31*	(1.18–9.29)	–	–
[a]STJ V6 (μV)	≤−20	≤−20	4.48**	(1.82–11.04)		
[b]TonV/TpV	≥0.55	≥0.56	7.76***	(3.18–18.90)	–	–
[c]θ(Tp|Tref) (°)			–	–	3.40***	(1.88–6.17)
[d]θ(Tinit|Tterm) (°)	≥38	≥35	–	–	1.93*	(1.08–3.47)

Modified from Rautaharju et al. [14], with permission
***Signifies $p < 0.001$; **$p < 0.01$;*$p < 0.05$ for hazard ratios
[a]STJ V6 is the J-point amplitude in V6 lead
[b]TonV/TpV is the ratio of spatial vector magnitudes at global T wave onset and T peak
[c]θ(Tp|Tref) is the spatial angle between Tpeak vector and the normal reference vector. (Tref) for spatial direction of repolarization
[d]θ(Tinit|Tterm) is the spatial angle between the mean initial and terminal T vectors from quintiles 1–3 and 4–5, respectively

in women. The presence of a positive, flat or less negative than −100 μV (−1 mm) TaVR amplitude in men and women with CVD calls for additional diagnostic evaluation and possibly stronger therapeutic measures for prevention of CHD death and SCD.

References

1. Agarwal SK, Heiss G, Rautaharju PM, Shahar E, Massing MW, Simpson Jr RJ. Premature ventricular complexes and the risk of incident stroke: the Atherosclerosis Risk in Communities (ARIC) study. Stroke. 2010;41(4):588–93.
2. Rautaharju P, Rautaharju F. Investigative electrocardiography in epidemiological studies and clinical trials. London: Springer; 2007. p. 1–289.
3. Bertoia ML, Triche EW, Michaud DS, Baylin A, Hogan JW, Neuhouser ML, Tinker LF, Van Horn L, Waring ME, Li W, Shikany JM, Eaton CB. Mediterranean and dietary approaches to stop hypertension dietary patterns and risk of sudden cardiac death in postmenopausal women. Am J Clin Nutr. 2014;99:344–51.
4. Bertoia ML, Allison MA, Manson JAE, Freiberg MS, Kuller LH, Solomon AJ, Limacher MC, Johnson KC, Curb JD, Wassertheil-Smoller S, Eaton CB. Risk factors for sudden cardiac death in post-menopausal women. Am Coll Cardiol. 2012;60:2674–82.
5. Rothman KJ, Greenland S. Modern epidemiology. 2nd ed. Philadelphia: Lippincott Williams and Wilkins; 1998.
6. Siscovick DS, Raghunathan TE, Rautaharju P, Psaty BM, Cobb LA, Wagner EH. Clinically silent electrocardiographic abnormalities and the risk of primary cardiac arrest among hypertensive patients. Circulation. 1996;94:1329–33.
7. Rautaharju PM, Zhou SH, Wong S, Calhoun HP, Berenson GS, Prineas R, Davignon A. Sex differences in the evolution of the electrocardiographic QT interval with age. Can J Cardiol. 1992;8:690–5.
8. Rautaharju PM, Warren J, Jain U, Wolf HK, Nielsen CL. Cardiac infarction injury score. An electrocardiographic coding scheme for ischemic heart disease. Circulation. 1981;64:249–56.
9. Rautaharju PM, Manolio TA, Siscovick D, Zhou SH, Gardin JM, Kronmal R, Furberg CD, Borhani NO, Newman A. The Cardiovascular Health Study Collaborative Research Group. Utility of new electrocardiographic models for left ventricular mass in older adults. Hypertension. 1996;28:8–15.
10. Siscovick DS, Raghunathan TE, Psaty BM, Koepsell TD, Wicklund KG, Lin X, Cobb L, Rautaharju PM, Copass MK, Wagner EH. Diuretic therapy for hypertension and the risk of primary cardiac arrest. N Engl J Med. 1994;330:1852–7.
11. Whitsel EA, Boyko EJ, Rautaharju PM, Raghunathan TE, Lin D, Pearce RM, Weinmann SA, Siscovick DS. Electrocardiographic QT interval prolongation and risk of primary cardiac arrest in diabetic patients. Diabetes Care. 2005;28:2045–7.
12. Straus SMJM, Kors JA, De Bruin ML, van der Hooft CS, Hofman A, Heeringa J MD, Deckers JW MD, PHD, Kingma JH, Sturkenboom MCJM, Stricker BHC, Witteman JCM. Prolonged QTc interval and risk of sudden cardiac death in a population of older adults. J Am Coll Cardiol. 2006;47:362–7.
13. Rautaharju PM, Zhang ZM, Warren J, Gregg RE, Haisty Jr WK, Kucharska-Newton AM, Rosamond WD, Soliman EZ. Electrocardiographic predictors of coronary heart disease and sudden cardiac deaths in men and women free from cardiovascular disease in the Atherosclerosis Risk in Communities (ARIC) study. J Am Heart Assoc. 2013;2(3):e000061. PubMed: PMID: 23723252.
14. Rautaharju PM, Zhang ZM, Haisty WK Jr, Kucharska-Newton AM, Rosamond WD, Soliman EZ. Electrocardiographic Repolarization-Related Predictors of Coronary Heart Disease and Sudden Cardiac Deaths in Men and Women with Cardiovascular Disease in the Atherosclerosis Risk in Communities (ARIC) Study. J Electrocardiol. 2015;48:101–11.

Chapter 7
The Utility of the Electrocardiogram in Left Ventricular Hypertrophy

Synopsis Classification accuracy of commonly used ECG-LVH criteria developed with echocardiographic left ventricular mass (Echo-LVM) as the ECG-independent standard is known to be limited. Two common reasons for the low accuracy of ECG-LVH are the large variability in ECG electrode placement and the large intra- and interreader variability of Echo-LVM used as a standard in developing ECG-LVH criteria. While the importance of the ECG in clinical diagnosis of left ventricular hypertrophy (LVH) has diminished, ECG-LVH has retained its importance as a predictor of adverse cardiac events in hypertensive women and men.

Limited data available with LVM estimated by magnetic resonance imaging (MRI-LVM) as the ECG-independent standard have confirmed the low classification accuracy of older ECG-LVH criteria. ECG-LVH accuracy is better in clinical populations with a higher prevalence of true LVH such as in valvular heart disease and hypertension referral clinics.

The risk for adverse cardiac events is increased for many ECG-LVH criteria, and the risk is highest for criteria which combine increased QRS voltage with repolarization abnormalities such as the LV strain pattern.

In hypertensive men and women regression of ECG-LVH has been associated with reduction of cardiovascular disease (CVD) events (CVD death, non-fatal MI or stroke). The utility of ECG-LVH for monitoring the effectiveness of hypertension intervention requires further research.

The availability of MRI has opened up a new phase for development of more satisfactory ECG criteria for LVH and for identification of improved predictors of adverse cardiac events. Consideration of gender and racial differences in future studies is recommended as a high priority item.

Abbreviations and Acronyms

CHD	Coronary heart disease
CHS	Cardiovascular heart study
CVD	Cardiovascular disease
ECG	Electrocardiogram electrocardiographic
HF	Heart failure

P.M. Rautaharju, *The Female Electrocardiogram: Special Repolarization Features, Gender Differences, and the Risk of Adverse Cardiac Events*,
DOI 10.1007/978-3-319-15293-6_7

IVCD	Indetermined-type left ventricular conduction defect
LBBB	Left bundle branch block
LIFE	Losartan intervention for endpoint reduction in hypertension
LV	Left ventricle
LVH	Left ventricular hypertrophy
LVM	LV mass
MC	Minnesota code
MESA	Multi-ethnic study of atherosclerosis
MRFIT	Multiple risk factor intervention trial
MRI	Magnetic resonance imaging
RBBB	Right bundle branch block
SCD	Sudden cardiac death

7.1 Introduction

Left ventricular hypertrophy (LVH) is an important predictor of adverse cardiac events including heart failure and cardiac mortality. For this reason ECG diagnosis of LVH is potentially important.

The main limitation of ECG-LVH in clinical diagnostic applications is the low sensitivity of ECG-LVH criteria evaluated with echocardiographic left ventricular mass (LVM) or LVM by magnetic resonance imaging (Echo-LVM and MRI-LVM, respectively) as independent standards. Classification accuracy of ECG-LVH is higher in clinical populations with higher prevalence of LVH such as hypertension referral clinic populations. The low sensitivity of ECG-LVH also limits its utility in comparing the LVH-prevalence in contrasting general populations in epidemiological studies. Various aspects of the application of ECG-LVH in epidemiological studies and clinical trials in were covered in the monograph of Rautaharju and Rautaharju [1].

The present chapter is primarily an upgrade of the monograph Chapter 7 cited above. New concepts are gradually emerging about the pathways of the evolution of hypertension to LVH and to systolic and diastolic heart failure (HF) [2, 3] including potential importance of eccentric LVH in diastolic HF. These developments have also helped in interpretation of the mechanisms of depolarization- and repolarization-related ECG abnormalities. The role of depolarization- and repolarization-related abnormalities as prognostic factors for adverse cardiac events will be considered in this chapter.

7.2 Cardiac Evolution from LVH to Heart Failure: Background Data

LVH is a common precursor and a strong independent risk factor for coronary heart disease (CHD), sudden cardiac death (SCD), HF and stroke. LVH in hypertensive heart disease produces structural myocardial changes including perivascular and myocardial fibrosis which precipitate diastolic dysfunction and create conditions for an arrhythmogenic substrate [3]. Although the prevalence of LVH is lower in women than in men, LVH becomes more common in post-menopausal women, and hypertension and LVH are stronger risk factors for stroke and HF in women than in men [2]. In the USA HF is associated with diastolic dysfunction in over one third of the patients with HF [3].

The traditional concept about the evolution of hypertensive heart disease postulates that LVH leads into concentric LVH and systolic HF and then progresses into diastolic HF. However, eccentric LVH is at least as common as concentric LVH according to echocardiographic data. Newer data evaluated by Drazner in his review article [4] suggest that concentric hypertrophy does not commonly progress to dilated cardiac failure after 5–7 years of follow-up in the absence of interval myocardial infarction and that LVH in hypertensive patients can evolve directly to dilated HF rather than first evolving into concentric hypertrophy.

The block diagram in Fig. 7.1 is a schematic of the pathway of the evolution of LVH into left ventricular dysfunction and HF. The bottom section of the diagram

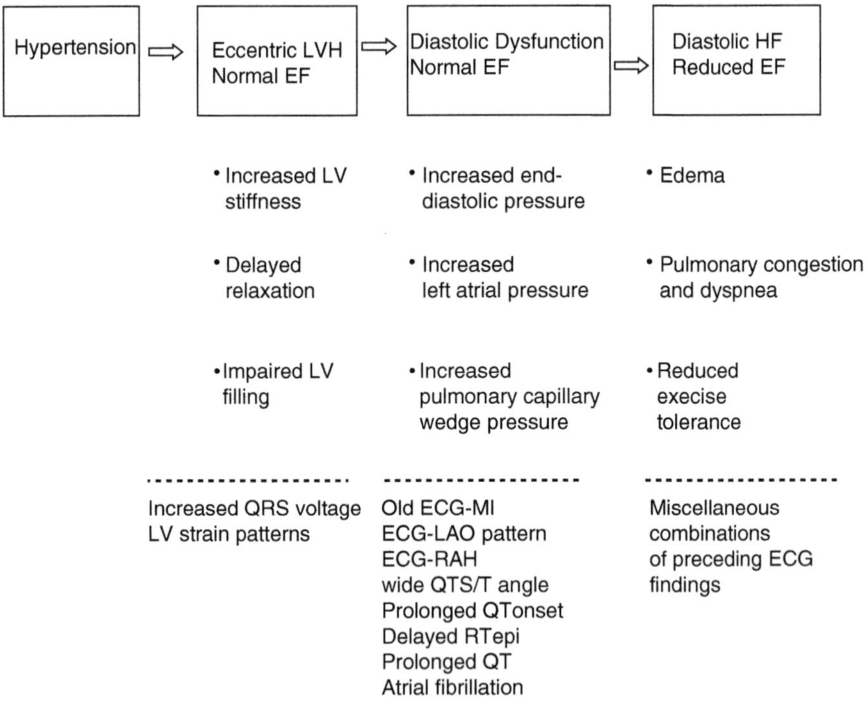

Fig. 7.1 A schematic showing ECG findings that can be expected (*bottom section*) in the evolution of hypertension to eccentric LVH, diastolic dysfunction and diastolic heart failure. *LV* left ventricular, *EF* ejection fraction, *MI* myocardial infarction, *LAO* left atrial overload, *RAH* right atrial hypertrophy, *RTepi* Epicardial repolarization time

lists ECG findings that can be expected in the course of the evolution. When early signs of diastolic dysfunction develop and the ejection fraction (EF) is still within normal limits, various ECG abnormalities that can be expected include transient AF, old ECG-MI, ECG signs of left atrial overload, wide QRS/T angle, delayed epicardial repolarization time (RTepi) and prolonged rate-adjusted QTend (QTea).

Frequently used ECG-LVH criteria in prognostic evaluation are listed in Table 7.1 as common reference for this chapter. The following criteria were included:

Table 7.1 Commonly used ECG criteria for left ventricular hypertrophy

Criteria [reference]	Variables	Criteria sets and limits
Sokolow-Lyon (SL) [5]	RV5 + SV1	1. SL >3,500 μV (men and women)
Minnesota Code MC 3.1 [6]	RI; RII; RIII; RaVL; RaVF; RV5	2A. Definite: R(I, II, III or AVF) >2,000 μV OR RaVL >1,200 μV OR RV5 > 2,600 μV
		2B. Borderline: 2A and (MC 4.1–4.3 or 5.1–5.3)
Minnesota Code MC 3.1+3.3	MC3.1 variables; RI; SL	3A. Definite: MC 3.1 OR SL >3 500 μV OR
		RI >1,500 μV (men and women)
		3B. Borderline: 3A and (MC 4.1–4.3 or 5.1–5.3)
Cornell voltage (CV) [7]	RaVL + SV3	4. CV >2,800 μV in men, >2,000 μV in women
Cornell product (CP) [8]	CV•QRSdur.	5. CP >240 μV.s (men and women)
Estes score ≥4 (ES4) [9] (possible LVH)	RV5; RV6; RI; RII; RIII; RaVR; RaVL; RaVF; SI; SII; SIII; SaVR; SaVL; SaVF QRSdur; LV strain†	6. RV5 or V6 ≥ 3,000 μV OR (R or S in any limb lead ≥3,000 μV) OR LV strain AND
		QRS >90 ms (men and women)
Estes score ≥5 (ES5) (definite LVH)	Variables above and P'V1	7. RV5/6 ≥ 3,000 μV OR SV5/6 ≥ 3,000 μV OR R or S in any limb lead ≥2,000 μV OR LV strain
Framingham score [9]	SL; RI; SIII; RaVL; SV1, V2; SL; LV strain	8. Borderline: SL criteria OR RaVL >1,100 μV OR (RI + SIII) ≥2,500 μV or RV5/6 ≥ 2,500 μV OR SV1/V2 ≥ 2,500 μV
		9. Definite: borderline criteria + LV strain
Perugia score [10]	SV3 + RaVL;	10. Men: RaVL + SV3 > 2,400 μV O RLV strain pattern or Romhilt-Estes score ≥5;
	Left ventricular strain;	
	Romhilt-Estes score	Women: RaVL + SV3 > 2,200 μV OR LV strain pattern OR Romhilt-Estes score ≥5;

LV left ventricle

†LV strain refers to downsloping ST segment with negative T wave in left lateral leads

Sokolow-Lyon [5], Minnesota Code [6], Cornell voltage [7], Cornell product [8], Estes score [9] and Perugia score [10].

Several ECG models have been introduced for prediction of left ventricular mass (LVM) on a continuous scale (Echo-LVM) [11–13] including a model derived in the Cardiovascular Heart Study (CHS) [13]. The algorithms for LVM from the CHS model are listed in Table 7.2 for normal ventricular conduction, anterior/lateral MI and ventricular conduction defects according to the Minnesota Code. Ranking of the best individual variables in each model according to their partial R-square values revealed that body weight was a dominant predictor in normal conduction, inferior myocardial infarction (MI) and right bundle branch block (RBBB), QRS duration in left bundle branch block (LBBB) and anterior and lateral MI and JV6 amplitude in indetermined-type ventricular conduction defect (ICVD) (not shown). The correlation between ECG-LVM from this model and Echo-LVM was 0.54 in women and 0.51 in men. In CHS study ECG-LVM and Echo-LVM had about equally strong associations with overt and subclinical disease and with risk factors for left ventricular hypertrophy.

7.3 Current Status of the Prognostic Utility of ECG-LVH

A representative example of prognostic evaluation results from a large sample of an urban population, the Copenhagen City Study [14] is shown in Fig. 7.2. Relative risk from 7-year follow-up for fatal and nonfatal ischemic heart disease events are displayed for five mutually exclusive hierarchic (from bottom to top) combinations of ECG abnormalities. There was no significant interaction between sex and ECG-LVH criteria and relative risks were determined for the combined group of men and women who were free of ischemic heart disease at the baseline. The risk was not significantly increased for high QRS voltage criteria (Minnesota Code (MC) 3.1/3.3). High QRS voltage combined with negative T waves (MC 5.1/5.3) had 1.89-fold increased risk and high QRS voltage combined with ST-T abnormalities (MC 4.1–4.3 and MC 5.1–5.3) had 3.62-fold risk. In addition, high voltage QRS plus ST depression and negative T wave had an age-adjusted relative risk increased 3.78-fold for myocardial infarction, 4.27-fold increased risk for ischemic heart disease and 3.75-fold increased risk for CVD (not shown).

Classification accuracy of commonly used ECG-LVH criteria is known to be limited. ECG-LVH criteria with best classification accuracy commonly do not have the highest predictive value. ECG-LVH criteria that combine high QRS voltage with ST-T abnormalities have generally the highest risk for adverse CVD events [15].

Two main factors have been suggested to be the reason for the limited classification accuracy of the commonly used ECG-LVH criteria: (1) Large variability in ECG electrode placement; and (2) Large variability in Echo-LVM estimation. In turn, two reasons have been suggested as the main reasons for the large variability of Echo-LVM estimation: (1) Echo-LVM estimate is based on LV wall thickness measurements with relatively large intra-and interreader variability,

Table 7.2 ECG-LVH and risk of adverse outcome events from the Framingham observational studies and two intervention studies

Study	Population	Endpoint	ECG-LVH criteria	Adjusted risk estimates (95 % CI)
Framingham [16]	28–62 years; CVD-free at baseline	Fatal and non-fatal CVD events	Cornell Voltage (CV) as a continuous variable	Baseline Quartile 4 vs. Quartile 1:
				Women: 3.29 (1.78–6.09)
				Men: 3.08 (1.87–5.07)
				CV decrease vs. no change during follow up
				Women: 0.56 (0.30–1.04)
				Men: 0.46 (0.28–0.54)
				CV increase vs. no change during follow up
				Women: 1.61 (0.94–2.84)
				Men: 1.86 (1.14–3.03)
Framingham [16]	28–62 years; CVD-free at baseline	Incident CVD (fatal and non-fatal)	Left ventricular (LV) strain	Baseline LV strain present vs. absent:
				Women: 2.47 (1 0.38–4.42)
				Men: 5.84 (3.55–9.62)
				LV strain improved vs. no change during follow up
				Women: 1.19 (0.56–2.49)
				Men: 0.45 (0.20–1.01)
				LV strain developed vs. no change during follow up
				Women: 2.02 (1.07–3.81)
				Men: 1.89 (1.05–3.40)
MRFIT [17]	Age 35–57, 12,866 men at high risk for CHD	CHD death,	Change in Sokolow-Lyon (SL) voltage	>900 μV decrease in SL: 1.2 (0.5–2.9)
			Change in Cornell voltage	>900 μV increase in SL: 1.9 (1.5–2.4)
				>400 μV decrease in CV: 1.3 (1.0–1.6)
				>400 μV increase in CV: 2.3 (1.8–3.1)
LIFE study [18]	Age 35–80; hypertensive men and women with ECG-LVH at baseline	CVD death, nonfatal MI or stroke	Sokolow-Lyon voltage	>1,050 μV decrease in SL: 0.80 (0.73–0.87)
			Cornell product (CP)	>105 μV.s decrease in CP: 0.78 (073–0.83)

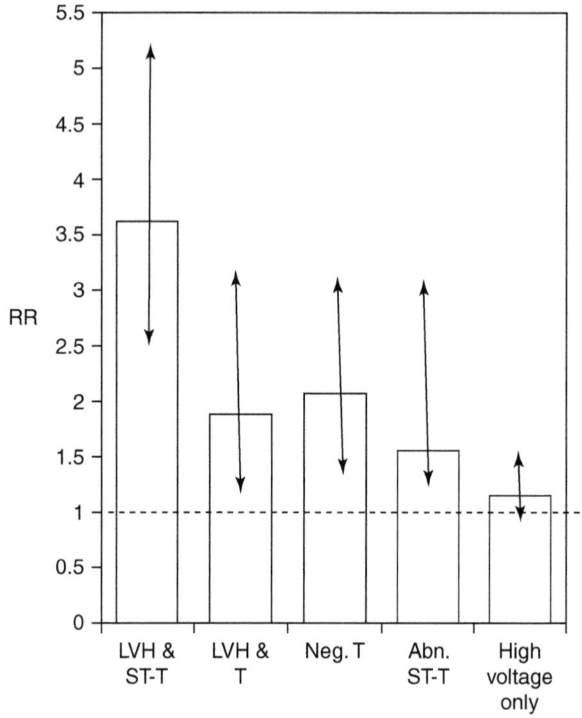

Fig. 7.2 Relative risk of 7-year fatal and nonfatal ischemic heart disease events in a large combined group of men and women free of ischemic heart disease at the baseline for ECG-LVH by Minnesota Code high voltage criteria with and without abnormal ST-T. The *double arrows* show the 95 % confidence intervals (From Table 4, Larsen et al. [14], with permission)

and (2) Geometric assumptions about LV shape. The combined effect of all these factors is the low classification accuracy of commonly used ECG-LVH criteria.

7.4 Prognostic Value of Progression Versus Regression of ECG-LVH

Data comparing progression vs. regression of ECG-LVH and risk of adverse outcome events are listed in Table 7.2 from the Framingham observational study and two intervention studies. Of particular interest in this context is the regression of ECG-LVH and the question whether regression of ECG-LVH can possibly be used as guidance for monitoring intervention on hypertension with ECG-LVH. The Framingham study [16] evaluated the risk for combined fatal and non-fatal CVD events for Cornell voltage (the first row in Table 7.2) and for Cornell voltage combined with LV strain pattern (the second row). Regression of Cornell voltage was associated with relative risk for CVD events reduced to approximately one half in women and in men although in women the 95 % CI was (0.30–1.04). Regression of Cornell voltage with LV strain pattern was associated with a reduced risk of CVD events in men but not in women.

The first of the two intervention studies in Table 7.2 is the Multiple Risk Factor Intervention Trial (MRFIT) [17]. The limits for significant increases and decreases in Sokolow-Lyon voltage and Cornell voltage were established as the upper 95 % limits for short-range daily variability. Decreased Sokolow-Lyon voltage was not associated with a reduction of the risk of CHD death, and reduction in Cornell voltage was actually associated with increased risk of CHD death.

The results from the Losartan Intervention for Endpoint Reduction in Hypertension (LIFE) were more encouraging [18, 19]. The reduction of ECG-LVH by Sokolow-Lyon voltage and by Cornell product (Cornell voltage*QRS duration) were both associated with decreased risk of CVD events (CVD death, non-fatal MI or stroke) in this study group of consisting of hypertensive men and women with ECG-LVH at baseline by the Sokolow-Lyon voltage or Cornell voltage criteria. Negative results in MRFIT compared to the LIFE study may reflect in part the fact that MRFIT intervention efforts failed, possibly due to aggressive hypertension control with diuretics used in the study or a combination of other factors. The second Losartan intervention study [19] documented that regression of ECG-LVH predicts regression of echocardiographic LVH thus lending support for the utility of ECG-LVH.

7.5 Classification Accuracy for ECG-LVH Criteria with Left Ventricular Mass by Magnetic Resonance Imaging as the Standard

MRI-LVM with three-dimensional multiplanar visualization of the heart, high blood-myocardial contrast, and high spatial-temporal resolution improves substantially the accuracy of LVM estimate as demonstrated by the MESA study [20]. Technical measurement error for LVM was established from a repeat variability study as 6 % of the mean LVM. Allometric formulation was derived to adjust LVM to height and weight in 1,746 MESA participants who were non-hypertensive and non-diabetic.

The overall classification accuracy for the older ECG-LVH criteria (Table 7.3) is best evaluated considering SEa, the sensitivity adjusted for equal level of specificity (95 %). SEa was quite low for all ECG-LVH criteria. Ignoring for the moment the MESA-specific criteria, SEa was highest for the Sokolow-Lyon criteria and Perugia Score (23 % for each). SEa was lowest for Romhilt-Estes Score ≥5 (9 %) and Framingham score (11 %).

Classification accuracy by ECG-LVH criteria can be expected higher in clinical conditions with higher prevalence of LVH such as in valvular heart disease. The studies that have used MRI as the ECG- independent standards are still limited. An example is the study of Buchner et al. [21]. These investigators evaluated 30 patients with aortic valve disease in comparison with 30 voluntaries. LVH was defined by MRI-LVM indexed to body surface area at 95th percentile in controls. Specificities (SP) and sensitivities (SE) for Cornell voltage and Sokolow-Lyon voltage were representative for the eight criteria evaluated. For Cornell criteria SE was 52 % and SP 87 %.

Table 7.3 Sensitivity and specificity, area under the ROC curve, sensitivity adjusted for specificity 0.95, total CVD event rates in no- LVH and LVH groups and multivariable-adjusted hazard ratio for ECG criteria in MESA study

	SE	SP	AUC	SEa	Event rate No LVH	Event rate LVH	Hazard ratio (95 % CI)	
Sokolow-Lyon	0.26	0.93	0.59	0.23	3.45	5.83*	1.26	(0.90–1.76)
Cornell voltage	0.15	0.97	0.56	0.15	3.55	6.55†	1.65	(1.03–2.63)
Minnesota Code 3.1	0.17	0.96	0.56	0.17	3.54	5.42*	1.15	(0.76–1.74)
Lewis index	0.23	0.89	0.56	0.17	3.43	5.34*	1.19	(0.87–1.60)
Gubner-Ungeleiter	0.14	0.95	0.54	0.13	3.55	5.32NS	1.01	(0.67–1.51)
Cornell voltage x QRS dur	0.15	0.97	0.54	0.17	3.48	8.57*	1.67	(1.09–2.54)
S-L voltage x QRS dur.	0.13	0.98	0.56	0.17	3.59	6.41NS	1.26	(0.71–2.23)
Isolated ischemic ST-T	0.11	0.97	0.54	0.13	3.51	7.89*	1.14	(0.73–1.76)
Framingham score (LV strain)	0.07	0.99	0.53	0.11	3.53	14.08*	2.04	(1.20–3.49)
Adjusted Framingham	0.15	0.97	0.56	0.17	3.55	6.51†	1.65	(1.03–2.63)
Romhilt-Estes score ≥4	0.16	0.97	0.56	0.17	3.5	7.51*	1.05	(0.69–1.61)
Romhilt-Estes score ≥5	0.06	0.99	0.52	0.09	3.54	13.59*	2.02	(1.15–3.54)
Perugia score	0.25	0.93	0.59	0.23	3.54	5.42*	1.15	(0.76–1.74
MESA criteria	0.40	0.90	0.65	0.35	3.34	5.92*	1.64	(1.21–2.21)

Adapted from Table 2, Jain et al. [20]

Multivariable-adjusted for age, BMI, gender, hypertension, diabetes, total and HDL cholesterol, pack-years of smoking, ethnicity, lipid and hypertensive medication, number of alcohol drinks per week, and physical activity

SE sensitivity %/100, *SP* specificity %/100, *AUC* area under the ROC curve, *SEa* 2*AUC-0.95 (Sensitivity adjusted for specificity 0.95), *Event Rate* CVD events per 10,000 person-days, *HR* hazard ratio

*Signifies P≤0.0005, †P≤0.005, and NS nonsignificant (P≤0.05) for z-test for proportions in event rates

For Sokolow-Lyon criteria SE was 57 % and SP 90 %. The overall classification accuracy was best for the Romhilt-Estes score ≥4: SE 86 % and SP 81 %. These classification accuracies for all of the ECG-LVH criteria are considerably higher than in non-valvular LVH. Another observation from that study was that T wave amplitudes in left lateral leads were mainly negative in eccentric LVH and positive in concentric LVH, consistent with the old concept of pressure vs. volume overload.

7.6 Risk for Composite CVD Events for ECG-LVH Criteria with MRI-LVM as the Standard

During a median follow-up of 4.8 years there were 307 CVD events among 4,938 MESA participants. The comparison of multivariable-adjusted hazard ratios for CVD events from those for the overall LVH classification accuracy according to sensitivity, specificity and AUC in Table 2 revealed some interesting contrasts (Table 7.3): Although classification accuracy was highest for the Sokolow-Lyon criteria and the Perugia score, HRs were not significant for either. In turn, HRs were highest for two LVH criteria with the lowest SEa, the Framingham LV strain and Romhilt-Estes Score ≥5, with HR = 2.04 each. Differences in classification accuracy do not mean much because for all practical purposes the classification accuracy for ECG-LVH criteria is too low. Differences in prognostic value for them convey more meaningful information.

The MESA study-specific ECG-LVH criterion obtained with a relatively minor modification of the Sokolow-Lyon criterion (RV5 plus sum of SV1 and SV2 instead of RV5 + SV1) with 40 % sensitivity at 90 % specificity. This is at least in part an expected result because these criteria were developed in this particular study population. The criteria need evaluation in a different populations. In any case, the use of MRI as a standard opens up a new phase for development of more satisfactory ECG criteria for LVH. The utility of the LVM models using MRI-LVM can be expected to improve from the models derived with Echo-LVM as the standard.

Heart failure is clinically often observed as the endpoint of LVH evolution over time in hypertension and other conditions inducing LVH. The pathways of evolution from CVD-free status to atrial fibrillation and heart failure and interactions in the vicious circle with each condition precipitating the other were covered in Chap. 5.

References

1. Rautaharju P, Rautaharju F. Investigative electrocardiography in epidemiological studies and clinical trials. London: Springer; 2007. p. 1–289.
2. Agabiti-Rosei E, Muiesan ML. Left ventricular hypertrophy and heart failure in women. J Hypertens Suppl. 2002;20:S34–8.
3. Gradman AH, Alfayoumi F. From left ventricular hypertrophy to congestive heart failure: management of hypertensive heart disease. Prog Cardiovasc Dis. 2006;48:326–41.
4. Drazner MH. The progression of hypertensive heart disease. Circulation. 2011;123:327–34.
5. Sokolow M, Lyon TP. The ventricular complex in left ventricular hypertrophy as obtained by unipolar precordial and limb leads. Am Heart J. 1949;37:161–86.
6. Blackburn H, Keys A, Simonson E, Rautaharju P, Punsar S. The electrocardiogram in population studies. A classification system. Circulation. 1960;21:1160–75.
7. Casale PN, Devereux RB, Kligfield P, Eisenberg RR, Miller DH, Chaudhary BS, Phillips MC. Electrocardiographic detection of left ventricular hypertrophy: development and prospective validation of improved criteria. J Am Coll Cardiol. 1985;6:572–80.
8. Molloy TJ, Okin PM, Devereux RB, Kligfield P. Electrocardiographic detection of left ventricular hypertrophy by the simple QRS voltage-duration product. J Am Coll Cardiol. 1992;20:1180–6.
9. Romhilt DW, Estes Jr EH. A point-score system for the ECG diagnosis of left ventricular hypertrophy. Am Heart J. 1968;75:252–8.
10. Verdecchia P, Schillaci G, Borgioni C, Ciucci A, Gattobigio R, Zampi I, Porcellati C. Prognostic value of new electrocardiographic method for diagnosis of left ventricular hypertrophy in essential hypertension. J Am Coll Cardiol. 1998;31:383–90.
11. Rautaharju PM, LaCroix AZ, Savage DD, Haynes S, Madans JH, Wolf HK, Hadden W, Keller J, Cornoni-Huntly J. Electrocardiographic estimate of left ventricular mass vs. radiographic

cardiac size and the risk of cardiovascular disease mortality in the epidemiologic follow-up study of the First National Health and Nutrition Examination Survey. Am J Cardiol. 1988;62:59–66.
12. Casale PN, Devereux RB, Alonso DR, Campo E, Kligfield P. Improved sex-specific criteria of left ventricular hypertrophy for clinical and computer interpretation of electrocardiograms: validation with autopsy findings. Circulation. 1987;75:565–72.
13. Rautaharju PM, Manolio TA, Siscovick D, Zhou SH, Gardin JM, Kronmal R, Furberg CD, Borhani NO, Newman A. For the Cardiovascular Health Study Collaborative Research Group. Utility of new electrocardiographic models for left ventricular mass in older adults. Hypertension. 1996;28:8–15.
14. Larsen CT, Dahlin J, Blackburn H, Scharling H, Appleyard M, Sigurd B, Schnohr P. Prevalence and prognosis of electrocardiographic left ventricular hypertrophy, ST segment depression and negative T-wave; the Copenhagen City Heart Study. Eur Heart J. 2002;23:315–24.
15. Rautaharju PM, Soliman EZ. Electrocardiographic left ventricular hypertrophy and the risk of adverse cardiovascular events: a critical appraisal. J Electrocardiol. 2014;90:1786–93.
16. Levy D, Salomon M, D'Agostino RB, Belanger AJ, Kannel WB. Prognostic implications of baseline electrocardiographic features and their serial changes in subjects with left ventricular hypertrophy. Circulation. 1994;90:1786–93.
17. Prineas RJ, Rautaharju PM, Grandits G, Crow R. For the MRFIT Research Group. Independent risk for cardiovascular disease predicted by modified continuous score electrocardiographic criteria for 6-year incidence and regression of left ventricular hypertrophy among clinically disease free men: 16 year follow-up for the Multiple Risk Factor Intervention Trial. J Electrocardiol. 2001;34:91–101.
18. Okin PM, Devereux RB, Jern S, Kjeldsen SE, Julius S, Nieminen MS, Snapinn S, Harris KE, Aurup P, Edelman JM, Wedel H, Lindholm LH, Dahlöf B. Regression of electrocardiographic left ventricular hypertrophy during antihypertensive treatment and the prediction of major cardiovascular events. JAMA. 2004;292:2343–9.
19. Okin PM, Devereux RB, Liu JE, Oikarinen L, Jern S, Kjeldsen SE, Julius S, Wachtell K, Nieminen MS, Dahlöf B. Regression of electrocardiographic left ventricular hypertrophy predicts regression of echocardiographic left ventricular mass: the LIFE study. J Hum Hypertens. 2004;18:403–9.
20. Jain A, Tandri H, Dalal D, Chahal H, Soliman EZ, Prineas R, Folsom AR, Lima JAC, Bluemke DA. Diagnostic and prognostic utility of electrocardiography for left ventricular hypertrophy defined by magnetic resonance imaging in relationship to ethnicity: the Multi-Ethnic Study of Atherosclerosis (MESA). Am Heart J. 2010;159:652–8.
21. Buchner S, Debl K, Haimerl J, Djavidani B, Poschenrieder F, Feuerbach S, Riegger GA, Luchner A. Electrocardiographic diagnosis of left ventricular hypertrophy in aortic valve disease: evaluation of ECG criteria by cardiovascular magnetic resonance. J Cardiovasc Magn Reson. 2009;11:18. doi:10.1186/1532-429X-11-18.

Chapter 8
Ventricular Conduction Defects in Women

Synopsis Ventricular conduction defects considered include left bundle branch block (LBBB), isolated right bundle branch block (RBBB), bifascicular block (RBBB with left anterior or left posterior fascicular block (LAFB and LPFB, respectively) and indetermined type ventricular conduction defect (IVCD).

In the Women's Health Initiative (WHI) study CHD mortality was increased for LBBB over threefold in CHD-free women and nearly threefold in women with CVD. The CHD mortality risk for isolated RBBB was increased significantly (1.62-fold) only in women with CVD as was the risk for IVCD (1.62-fold increase). The risk for all-cause mortality was increased significantly in women with CVD at baseline for LBBB (1.43-fold) and for bifascicular block (2.69-fold) but not in any other subgroup by bundle branch block category and CVD status.

The risk for incident HF was evaluated in another WHI study. Compared to women with no bundle branch block, LBBB and IVCD were strong predictors of incident HF. RBBB was not a significant predictor of incident HF in multivariable-adjusted risk model but RBBB combined with LAFB was a strong predictor. QRS duration was an independent predictor of incident HF only in LBBB, with more pronounced risk for QRS ≥140 ms than for <140 ms. QRS nondipolar voltage (RNDPV) was an independent predictor in both RBBB and LBBB and in LBBB in addition, spatial QRS/T angle and ST J-point depression in aVL were independent predictors.

Repolarization abnormalities in bundle branch blocks are generally considered as strictly secondary to increased QRS duration and altered spatial sequence of depolarization and consequently clinically of little diagnostic or prognostic utility. This chapter covers more recent studies which demonstrate that repolarization abnormalities also in bundle branch blocks are important predictors of increased risk of coronary heart disease (CHD) and cardiovascular disease (CVD) mortality and adverse events such as heart failure (HF).

Abbreviations and Acronyms

ARIC	Arteriosclerosis research in communities study
CHD	Coronary heart disease
HF	Heart failure

P.M. Rautaharju, *The Female Electrocardiogram: Special Repolarization Features, Gender Differences, and the Risk of Adverse Cardiac Events*, DOI 10.1007/978-3-319-15293-6_8

HR	Hazard ratio
IVCD	Indetermined type ventricular conduction defect
LAFB	Left anterior fascicular block
LBBB	Left bundle branch block
LPFB	Left posterior fascicular block
RBBB	Right bundle branch block
RNDPV	QRS nondipolar voltage
Rp	R wave peak in the spatial QRS vector magnitude function
Tp	T wave peak in the spatial T vector magnitude function
VCD	Ventricular conduction defect
WHI	Women's Health Initiative
$\Theta(R_m \mid T_m)$	Spatial angle between the mean QRS and ST-T vectors
Θ(Rp|Tp)	Spatial angle between the peak QRS and peak T vectors
Θ(Tinit|Tterm)	Spatial angle between the initial and terminal T vectors

8.1 Introduction

Repolarization abnormalities in bundle branch blocks (BBB) are generally considered as strictly secondary to increased QRS duration and altered spatial sequence of depolarization and clinically of little diagnostic or prognostic utility. More recent studies covered in this chapter have demonstrated that repolarization abnormalities in BBB are important predictors of increased risk of coronary heart disease (CHD) and cardiovascular disease (CVD) mortality and adverse events such as heart failure (HF). BBBs considered in this chapter include left and right BBB (LBBB and RBBB, respectively, indetermined type ventricular conduction defect (IVCD) and bifascicular block (RBBB combined with left anterior fascicular block (LAFB) or left posterior fascicular block (LPFB)). The prevalence and the mortality risk for ventricular conduction defects from epidemiological studies before 2007 was covered previously [1].

BBBs induce various degrees of repolarization changes ranging from relatively minor, mainly terminal repolarization changes in RBBB to profound repolarization changes in LBBB.

8.2 Ventricular Conduction Defects, Repolarization Abnormalities and Mortality Risk in Women

New information about the mortality risk and the risk of incident heart failure (HF) specifically in women has emerged from the Women's Health Initiative study reports [2, 3]. The mortality risk findings in bundle branch blocks will be addressed here first.

In the report of Zhang et al. [2] 66,450 WHI women were followed for 14 years. The risk for CVD death and deaths from all causes was evaluated for women with and without CVD at the baseline. Table 8.1 reproduced from Table 2 of Zhang et al. summarizes the results for LBBB and RBB. There were 714 women with LBBB at baseline and RBBB was coded in 832 women. Focusing on risk models multivariable-adjusted for demographic and clinical risk factors, the highlights of the findings were the following:

The risk for CHD-death for LBBB was increased 2.17-fold for women free from cardiovascular disease (CVD) and nearly threefold (HR 2.92, CI 2.08–4.08) for women with CVD. The risk for all-cause mortality was increased significantly for LBBB in women with CVD at baseline (HR 1.43, CI 1.11–1.83); the risk for all-cause mortality was not significantly increased in any other subgroup by bundle branch block category and CVD status. For isolated RBBB the risk for CHD death was significantly increased only in women with CVD (HR 1.62, CI 1.08–2.43). For RBBB combined with LAFB in women with CVD the risk. The risk for CHD death was increased over threefold (HR 3.09, CI 1.26–7.58) and over twofold for total mortality (HR 2.69, CI 1.55–4.67). And for IVCD the risk for CHD death was increased significantly for women with CVD (HR 2.52, CI 1.34–4.75).

8.2.1 Repolarization Abnormalities and Mortality Risk in Ventricular Conduction Defects

In the above study [2] QRS duration was entered simultaneously with QRS|T angle and other repolarization parameters as covariates. QRS duration was not a significant independent predictor of CHD death. None of the repolarization parameters

Table 8.1 Hazard ratios with 95 % confidence intervals for coronary heart disease death for bundle branch block categories by baseline cardiovascular disease status

CVD status	Category	Event rate	Univariate	Multivariate[a]
CVD-free	No BBB	894/52,663(1.7 %)	HR = 1	HR = 1
	LBBB	24/408 (5.9 %)	2.40 (1.60–3.61)	2.17 (1.37–3.43)
	RBBB	21/534 (3.9 %)	1.68 (1.09–2.59)	1.31 (0.77–2.23)
CVD	No BBB	597/12,048 (5.0 %)	HR = 1	HR = 1
	LBBB	48/306 (15.7 %)	2.85 (2.12–3.82)	2.92 (2.08–4.08)
	RBBB	27/298 (9.1 %)	1.60 (1.09–2.36)	1.62 (1.08–2.43)
	IVCD	10/73 (13.7 %)	2.72 (1.46–5.08)	2.52 (1.34–4.75)
	RBBB & LAFB	5/31 (16.1 %)	2.87 (1.19–6.92)	3.09 (1.26–7.58)

From Zhang et al. [2], with permission

Abbreviations: *BBB* bundle branch block, *CVD* cardiovascular disease, *HR* hazard ratio, *RBBB* right bundle branch block, *LBBB* left bundle branch block, *IVCD* intraventricular conduction defect of indetermined type, *LAFB* left anterior fascicular block

[a]Multivariate risk model adjusted for age, ethnicity, body mass index, smoking status, hypertension, diabetes mellitus, cancer, previous stroke, history of cardiovascular disease, hypercholesterolemia, emphysema, family history of coronary heart disease, systolic blood pressure, heart rate, and study component/arm groups (hormone therapy/dietary modification/calcium and vitamin D)

were significant independent ECG predictors of CHD death in RBBB. In LBBB, ST J-point depression in aVL was a markedly strong independent predictor of CHD mortality with an over fivefold increased risk in fully-adjusted risk model. This was the first study which evaluated mortality risk associated with repolarization parameters as covariates in LBBB and RBBB.

8.3 Independent Predictors for Heart Failure in Left Bundle Branch Block and Right Bundle Branch Block

HF risk data for independent ECG predictors of HF in CHD-free women and in women with CVD at baseline reproduced in Table 8.2 from the report of Zhang et al. [3] reveals some interesting associations for HF risk in multivariable-adjusted models.

QRS nondipolar voltage (RNDPV) was a strong independent predictor for HF in RBBB (HR 3.31, CI 1.09–10.0) and in LBBB (HR 1.89, CI 1.05–3.41). RNDPV was the only significant independent predictor for HF in RBBB but several other ECG variables were independent predictors in LBBB with an approximately two-fold increase risk for all. QRS duration was an independent predictor of incident HF in LBBB, with more pronounced risk for QRS ≥140 ms than for QRS <140 ms.

Table 8.2 Significant independent ECG predictors of incident heart failure in women for baseline LBBB and RBBB

	Test group[a] cutoff	Model 1[b]	Model 2[b]	Model 3[b]
LBBB (n 680)				
Heart rate/min	>75	1.94 (1.22–3.09)	1.84 (1.13–2.98)	2.01 (1.09–3.70)
[c]RNDVP (μV)	≥107	1.83 (1.15–2.93)	1.64 (1.00–2.47)	1.89 (1.05–3.41)
[d]STJ aVL (μV)	<–25	2.60 (1.67–4.06)	1.85 (1.10–3.12)	1.89 (1.05–3.41)
QRS dur. (ms)	≥140	1.77 (1.12–2.79)	1.59 (1.00–2.58)	1.87 (1.01–3.46)
[e]$\Theta(R_m\|T_m)$ (°)	≥63	2.01 (1.26–3.19)	1.41 (0.80–2.47)	1.97 (1.05–3.41)
RBBB (n 740)				
RNDVP (μV)	≥112	2.53 (1.24–5.19)	2.81 (1.16–5.34)	3.31 (1.09–10.0)[b]
QRS dur. (ms)	≥140	1.34 (0.66–2.72)	1.14 (0.55–2.37)	1.00 (0.37–2.74)

Modified from Zhang et al. [3] (Table 4), with permission

[a]Quintile 5 with quintiles 1–4 as the reference group except QRS ≥140 ms vs. QRS120-139 ms for LBBB and RBBB

[b]Model 1: Unadjusted single ECG variable risk model (included heart rate, QRS duration, QTrr, QRS/T angle, RNDVP, ST amplitude at J-point in leads of aVR, aVL, V1 and V6, and T wave amplitude in the leads of aVR, aVL, V1 and V6, separately); Model 2: Significant predictors in Model 1 entered simultaneously and each adjusted for the other ECG covariates; Model 3: ECG variables in Model 2 entered simultaneously and adjusted for demographic and clinical factors listed in the footnote of Table 2

[c]RNDPV = QRS nondipolar voltage from singular value decomposition

[d]STJ = J-point amplitude

[e]$\Theta(R_m|T_m)$ = spatial angle between the mean QRS and T vectors

Wide spatial angle (>65°) between the mean QRS and ST-T vectors ($\Theta(R_m|T_m)$) was a significant predictor of HF in LBBB as was ST J-point depression >25 μV in aVL, with an approximately twofold increased risk for both

8.4 QRS/T Angle and Heart Failure Risk in Bundle Branch Blocks in Women Compared to Men

In a recent report from the Arteriosclerosis Risk in Communities (ARIC) study the risk for new-onset HF in women and men was evaluated [4]. The report focused specifically on the impact of $\Theta(Rp|Tp)$, the spatial angle between peak QRS and peak T vectors on HF risk. QRS/T angle was dichotomized using upper quartile limits as cut points for each bundle branch group. Using men and women with no bundle branch and QRS/T angle quartiles 1–3 as the reference group HF risk for wide QRS/T angle was increased 75 % for IVCD (HR 1.75, CI (1.19–2.57)) and close to threefold for LBBB (HR 2.87, CI (1.19–2.57)). RBBB was not significantly associated with HF risk at any level of QRS/T angle. The results were consistent across subgroups by gender. For pooled bundle branch group including LBBB, IVCD and RBBB with LAFB or LPFB but excluding isolated RBBB, HF risk was increased over twofold (HR 2.29, CI 1.80–2.92).

QRS/T angle in women with LBBB combined with IVCD was wider than in men (138° vs. 119°) although the angle was narrower in women with no BBB than in men (61° vs. 75°). Additional regression analyses performed (not shown) revealed that 58 % of the gender difference in QRS/T angle (11° of 19° wider angle in women) was associated with a more pronounced increase in QRS duration in women than in men (in women 86 ms in No-BBB, 120 ms in BBB, in men 91 ms in No-BBB, 133 ms in BBB). This indicates that 58 % of the more pronounced increase in QRS/T angle in women is secondary to more pronounced QRS duration increase, and that the remaining 42 % (8°) is due to primary repolarization abnormalities which existed before BBB developed.

Hazard ratios for heart failure for women and men with and without bundle branch block by dichotomized spatial QRS/T angle are listed in Table 8.3. The table shows that the HF risk levels in women are comparable to those in men. Using women and men with no bundle branch block and normal QRS/T angle as the reference group, HF risk for women with BBB and normal QRS/T angle was increased twofold (HR 2.03, CI (1.36–3.02)) and for men increased by 45 % (HR 1.44, CI (1.05–1.95)). There was a further substantial increase in HF risk in women and men with bundle branch block and wide QRS/T angle. For women the risk was well over fourfold (HR 4.85, CI 2.72–8.67) and for men over threefold (HR 3.17, CI 2.15–4.68).

Frontal plane QRS/T angle defined as the absolute difference in frontal plane QRS and T axis from GE-Marquette ECG report was equally strong predictor as the spatial QRS/T angle. Furthermore, in evaluation of independent predictors of HF risk it was found that the presence of a positive T wave amplitude in aVR lead was as potent predictor of AF as the QRS/T angles.

Table 8.3 Incidence rates and hazard ratios heart failure for women and men with and without bundle branch block by QRS/T Angle

[a]BBB/QRS/T group	HF incidence/1,000 person-years	Hazard ratio[b] (95 % CI)		
	Women	Men	Women	Men
No-BBB/ QRS/T < 75th %	5.9	7.6	1.00 (ref)	1.00 (ref)
No-BBB/ QRS/T ≥ 75th %	11.1	15.9	**1.45 (1.27–1.65)**	**1.64 (1.42–1.89)**
BBB/ QRS/T < 75th %	16.0	17.3	**2.03 (1.36–3.02)**	**1.44 (1.05–1.95)**
BBB/ QRS/T ≥ 75th %	27.2	36.1	**4.85 (2.72–8.67)**	**3.17 (2.15–4.68)**

Modified from Table 3, Zhang et al. [4], with permission

[a]*BBB* bundle branch block, test group cut points for spatial QRS/T angle at 75th percentile in No-BBB group ≥95° for men and ≥77° for women and in BBB group ≥134° for men and ≥145° for women

[b]Risk model adjusted for demographic and clinical variables (age, race, region of residence, body mass index, systolic blood pressure, smoking status, education, hypertension, diabetes mellitus, cardiovascular disease status, ratio of total cholesterol/high-density lipoprotein, blood glucose, serum creatinine, and QRS duration at baseline)

8.5 Spatial Distributions of Rpeak and Tpeak Vectors in No-BBB, LBBB and RBBB

Spatial distributions of Rpeak and Tpeak vectors in No-BBB, LBBB and RBBB are shown in Figs. 8.1, 8.2 and 8.3. In these frontal plane projections of a rhombic 3-D reference frame introduced in Chap. 3, the letters in the labels refer to the six principal directions: L = Left; R = Right; I = Inferior; S = Superior; A = Anterior; and P = Posterior. The letters in acronyms for rhombic faces are in order of dominance of principal axis: ILA = Inferior-Left-Anterior, etc.

Spatial Rpeak (Rp) and Tpeak (Tp) vector directions in No-BBB in Fig. 8.1 show that Rp vector direction is Left (L) in 58 % and in 29 % Inferior-Left-Anterior (ILA). Rp and Tp distributions overlap to a large decree. Figure 8.1 shows that in comparison to Rp distribution 44 % of the Tp vectors have shifted from direction L to ILA or Anterior-Left (AL). The computed spatial angle between Rp and Tp vectors, Θ(Rp|Tp), is 44° in No-BBB group.

In LBBB the distributions of Rp and Tp vectors differs substantially from those in No-BBB as shown in Fig. 8.2. The figure shows a pronounced posterior-left shift of Rp vector directions in No-BBB, with 97 % of Rp vectors in direction Posterior-Left (PL). Tp vectors, in turn, have shifted to the opposite direction compared with Rp vectors, with 78 % of Tp vectors have shirted to Anterior-Right (AR). As a consequence, the computed Θ(Rp|Tp) is 153°.

Rpeak (Rp) and Tpeak (Tp) vector directions in RBBB are shown in Fig. 8.3. Rp and Tp distributions differ little from those in No-BBB in Fig. 8.1 but the differences from Rp and Tp distributions are profound compared with those for LBBB in Fig. 8.2. Rp and Tp distributions in RBBB overlap as did the Rp and Tp distributions

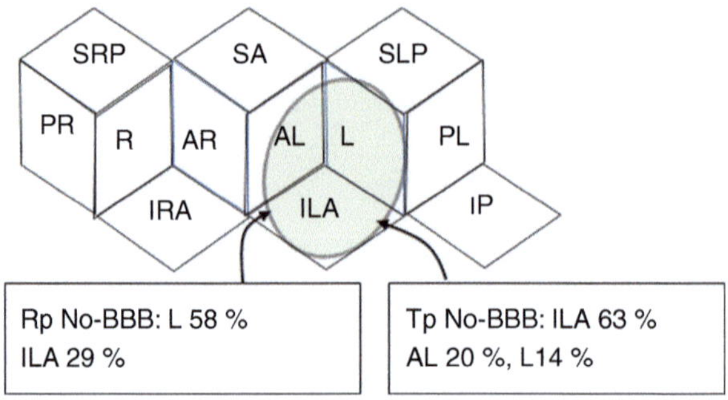

Fig. 8.1 Spatial Rpeak (*Rp*) and Tpeak (*Tp*) vector directions in No-BBB. Rp vectors are directed to the left (*L*) in 58 % and to inferior-left anterior (*ILA*) in 29 %. In comparison with Rp vector directions, only 14 % of Tp vectors remain directed to L while 44 % of them have shifted to ILA or anterior-left (*AL*). The computed spatial angle between Rp and Tp vectors, Θ(Rp|Tp), in No-BBB is 44°

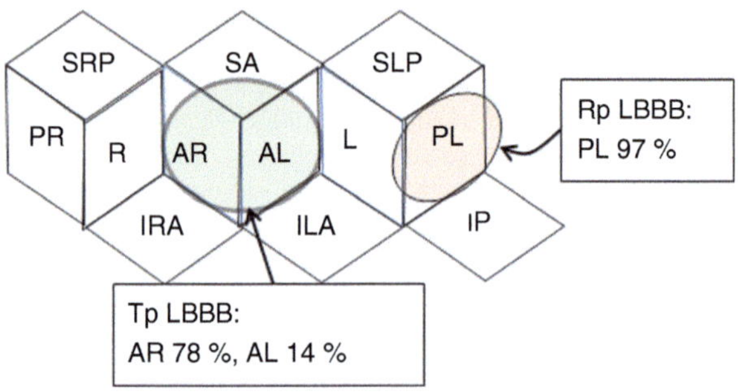

Fig. 8.2 Spatial Rpeak (*Rp*) and Tpeak (*Tp*) vector directions in LBBB. Rp vectors are directed to posterior-left in 97 % indicating a pronounced posterior-left shift from Rp vector directions in No-BBB in Fig. 8.1. Tp vectors in LBBB in contrast to Rp vectors, have shifted in opposite direction with 78 % of them shifted to anterior-right (*AR*). This suggests a widening of Θ(Rp|Tp), the spatial angle between the Rp and Tp vectors. The computed Θ(Rp|Tp) in LBBB is 153° compared to 44° in No-BBB

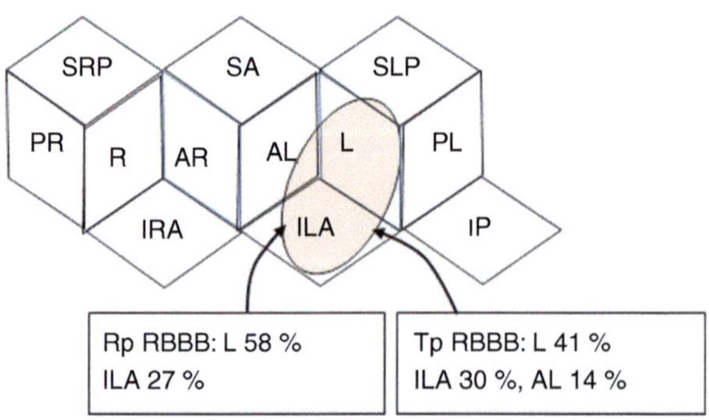

Fig. 8.3 Spatial Rpeak (*Rp*) and Tpeak (*Tp*) vector directions in RBBB. Rp vectors are directed to the left (*L*) in 58 % and to inferior-left-anterior (*ILA*) in 27 %. The distributions of Rp and Tp vectors overlap except that more Rp vectors are in direction L than Tp vectors (58 % vs. 41 %, respectively) and 14 % of Tp vectors have shifted to anterior-left (*AL*). The computed Θ(Rp|Tp) in RBBB is 44° as in No-BBB

in No-BBB. Figure 8.3 shows that more Rp vectors are in direction L than Tp vectors (58 % vs. 41 %, respectively) and 14 % of Tp vectors have shifted to anterior-left (AL). The computed Θ(Rp|Tp) in RBBB is 44° as in No-BBB.

8.6 The Mechanism for High Risk for Left Bundle Branch Block

Risk data above have consistently shown a high mortality risk for LBBB. The prevalence of bundle branch blocks increase with older age and hypertension and it has been suggested that bundle branch blocks including RBBB are a manifestation of the general degenerative process of the cardiovascular system including the heart [6]. However, cardiac excitation and repolarization in LBBB differs from RBBB.

Large spatial angle between Rp and Tp vectors has been documented to be associated with increased risk for CVD morbidity and mortality such as incident HF and CHD mortality as was documented in Sects. 8.3 and 8.4 above. The spatial angle between Rp and Tp vectors in LBBB was 153°. In RBBB, in contrast to LBBB, the spatial angle between Rp and Tp vectors was 44°. These findings may account for the higher risk of adverse outcomes in LBBB than in RBBB. Θ(Rp|Tp) in LBBB was 153°. While Rp direction represents the spatial direction of excitation gradient (RTgrad) at time point when the largest number of ventricular myocytes are depolarizing, temporal repolarization time gradient vector (RTgrad) direction is diametrically opposite to the direction of Tp vector. Thus the spatial angle between ETgrad and RTgrad vectors in LBBB is (180–153) or 27°. This implies that the direction of repolarization sequence is concordant with respect to the direction of excitation sequence. In concordant repolarization in LBBB QT will prolong in proportion to QRS duration. QRS duration has been found in women to be an independent predictor of incident HF in LBBB, with more pronounced risk at QRS ≥140 ms than at <140 ms [3].

In addition, the difference (QTea-QTpa) interval which represents global RT dispersion is prolonged to 107 ms in LBBB and to 94 ms in RBBB compared to normal reference QTea-QTpa (89 ms). This corresponds to the 17 ms QTea prolongation in LBBB and 6 ms prolongation in RBBB.

The main feature of LBBB repolarization is that repolarization is progressively delayed in proportion to delay in excitation. Delayed repolarization sequence changes the normally reversed repolarization sequence to a concordant sequence with respect depolarization sequence. The observed increased depolarization delay across the left ventricle in LBBB increases the dyssynchrony of ventricular contraction which is considered as the primary mechanism for abnormal cardiac function and the risk for HF. Electrophysiological data, although limited, suggest that dyssynchrony of repolarization and left ventricular repolarization prolonging left ventricular isovolumic relaxation period is also an important contributing factor for abnormal cardiac function and the risk for HF [5]. This postulate is consistent with the observed profound increase in the risk for HF for widened QRS/Tangle [4].

8.7 Right Bundle Branch Block as a Mortality Predictor

8.7.1 The Framingham Study

Most previous studies have found no significant association for RBBB with adverse cardiac outcome events. In a 1980 report from the Framingham study 70 persons developed a new RBBB during 18 year follow-up [6]. Although most of them were hypertensive, overt clinical events were uncommon at the initial appearance of RBBB. However, the subsequent incidence of CHD was two and one-half times higher and that of HF four times higher and CVD mortality almost three times greater than in matched control subjects without RBBB. A remarkable finding in the study was that only 21% remained free from clinically apparent CVD abnormalities. Another intriguing finding was that QRS duration was 130 ms or in incident RBBB. Furthermore, the frontal plane QRS axis between −45° and −90° (i.e. RBBB with left axis deviation).is This subgroup evidently had RBBB combined with left anterior fascicular block and most likely had additional repolarization abnormalities.

8.7.2 The Copenhagen City Heart Study

The Copenhagen report has brought new evidence about the prognostic importance of RBBB [7]. In this large representative urban population the prevalence of RBBB was higher in men than in women (1.4 % vs. 0.5 %, $P<0.001$) as has been generally found in other studies. RBBB was identified in 119 men and 47 women. Among the 10 629 participants free from RBBB at the first examination, 51 (33 men and 18 women) developed RBBB during the median 20.5 year follow-up. Prevalent and incident RBBB were associated with higher age, male gender and higher blood pressure but the association with other CVD risk factors was not consistent. The authors infer that RBBB when seen in patients free from CVDs should not be regarded as a marker of the cumulative effect of traditional cardiovascular risk factors causing CHD but as a marker of progressive degenerative disease. The authors also note that the higher prevalence of RBBB in men compared with women was not caused by differences in risk factor distribution and remains largely unexplained.

From the group with RBBB at baseline 107 men and 38 women died. Results from survival analyses of different outcomes in men, women and pooled gender groups indicated that hazard ratios were comparable in men and women with the exception that significant association between RBBB and myocardial infarction was observed in women (HR 2.79, CI (1.50–5.22)) but the association was not significant for men. The authors note that this may have been a chance result finding because of multiple comparisons. Overall the increased mortality was caused by increased cardiovascular mortality (HR 1.87, CI 1.48–2.36).

References

1. Rautaharju P, Rautaharju F. Investigative electrocardiography in epidemiological studies and clinical trials. London: Springer; 2007. p. 1–289.
2. Zhang ZM, Rautaharju PM, Soliman EZ, Manson JE, Cain ME, Martin LW, Bavry AA, Mehta L, Vitolins M, Prineas RJ. Mortality risk associated with bundle branch blocks and related repolarization abnormalities (from the Women's Health Initiative [WHI]). Am J Cardiol. 2012;110:1489–95.
3. Zhang ZM, Rautaharju PM, Soliman EZ, Manson J-A, Martin LW, Perez M, Vitolins M, Prineas RJ. Different patterns of bundle branch blocks and the risk of incident heart failure in the Women's Health Initiative (WHI) Study. Circ Heart Fail. 2013;6:655–61.
4. Zhang ZM, Rautaharju PM, Prineas RJ, Loehr L, Rosamond W, Soliman EZ. Usefulness of electrocardiographic QRS/T angles with versus without bundle branch blocks to predict heart failure (From the Atherosclerosis Risk in Communities [ARIC] Study). Am J Cardiol. 2014;114:412–8.
5. Zhu TG, Patel C, Martin S, Quan X, Ying Wu Y, Burke JF, Chernick M, Kowey PR, Yan GX. Ventricular transmural repolarization sequence: its relationship with ventricular relaxation and role in ventricular diastolic function. Eur Heart J. 2009;30:372–80.
6. Schneider JF, Thomas HE, Kreger BE, McNamara PM, Sorlie P, Kannel WB. Newly acquired right bundle-branch block: the Framingham Study. Ann Intern Med. 1980;92:37–44.
7. Bussink BE, Holst AG, Jespersen L, Deckers JW, Jensen GB, Prescott E. Right bundle branch block: prevalence, risk factors, and outcome in the general population: results from the Copenhagen City Heart Study. Eur Heart J. 2013;34:138–46.

Chapter 9
ST-T Waveform Features, QT and Mortality Risk

Synopsis QT interval is the repolarization time (RT) of the ventricular region repolarized last. Epicardial and endocardial RT (RTepi and RTendo) represent regional RTs and QT subintervals. Based on these ECG measures of repolarization a working model was constructed to account for gender differences in the waveform of the ST and the durations of QT and QT subintervals.

Normal and abnormal repolarization patterns are generated by ion channel currents which modulate regional action potential durations (APD) and waveforms. In normal men the transient outward potassium current (I_{to}) plays an important role in generating the characteristic male ST-T waveform. Increased Ito shifts the ST segment dome to a higher potential level, reduces APD, enhances activation of the delayed rectifiers ($I_{Ks,}I_{Kr}$) and promotes faster repolarization. Action potential phase 2 and phase 3 slopes decrease (become more negative) generating the asymmetric T waveform in males with upsloping 'U-shaped' ST segment with reduced convexity and tall T wave.

Epicardial and endocardial action potential difference at phase 2 in women in contrast to men, is minimal so that STJ-point elevation is absent and ST segment is flat. The convexity of the J-Tp segment is high. Potassium channel subunit Kir2.3 levels in females at epicardium have been found to be lower than at endocardium. Kir2.3 mediates cardiac inward rectifier I_{K1}. There are several expected results from lower Kir2.3 level. RTepi is prolonged more than RTendo. Rate-adjusted QTpeak (QTpa) prolongs. The interval from Tpeak (Tp) to the inflection point at T wave downstroke (Txd) representing crossmural dispersion of left ventricular repolarization (TpTxd interval) increases and also QT increases if TpTe remains unchanged or increases (by reduced IK1 prolonging phase 3 at basal regions normally repolarized last).

The gender difference in QT is due to QT shortening in adolescent boys and QT remains shorter in men than in women through adulthood. Testosterone modulates the main repolarizing current (L-typeCa^{2+}) at phase 2 and the primary repolarizing current (I_{Ks}) during phase 3, shortening APD and QT.

ECG measures of deviant repolarization are clinically important predictors of adverse outcome events, including various angular measures of the spatial direction of deviant repolarization. Sex differences in ion channel currents modulating action

P.M. Rautaharju, *The Female Electrocardiogram: Special Repolarization Features, Gender Differences, and the Risk of Adverse Cardiac Events*,
DOI 10.1007/978-3-319-15293-6_9

potential durations are not only of interest from the perspective of electrophysiological mechanisms to elucidate their mechanism but they have practical clinical implications as described in previous chapters.

Abbreviations Acronyms and Ion Channel Current Labels

AF	Atrial fibrillation
APD	Action potential duration
CHD	Coronary heart disease
CVD	Cardiovascular disease
HF	Heart failure
ICaL	Inward calcium current with long-lasting activated state
ICaT	Transient inward calcium current
IK1	Potassium current in inward rectifier ion channel
IKACh	Inward potassium current through ACh-activated K^+ channel.
IKr	Rapidly activating outward rectifying potassium current
IKs	Slowly activating outward rectifying potassium current
IKur	Ultrarapidly activating outward rectifying potassium current
INa	Inward sodium current
Ito	Transient outward potassium current
LGIC	Ligand-gated ion channel ion channel proteins which bind a chemical messenged (ligand) such as neurotransmitter and open a channel to ion transport through the membrane
NCX	Sodium-calcium exchange protein that removes 1 Ca^{2+} from inside cell in exchange of 3 Na^+
SA	Sino-atrial node
SCD	Sudden cardiac death

9.1 Introduction

Consideration of cardiac ion channel currents and the factors that modulate them is of utmost importance for the understanding of the QT interval and other repolarization features. A variety of labels have been used in electrophysiological literature for ion currents. In this chapter the labels for ion currents follow the terminology used by Grant is his extensive review [1]. Ion currents are activated and inactivated at various phases of action potential. Figure 9.1 adapted from the review by Nattel and Carlson [2] shows ion currents that generate normal ventricular action potential upstroke (phase 0), overshoot and notch (phase1), slow phase of repolarization (plateau or phase 2), fast phase of repolarization (phase 3) and the resting potential (phase 4). Of main interest in this context are the ion currents involved in modifying action potential duration (APD) and waveform.

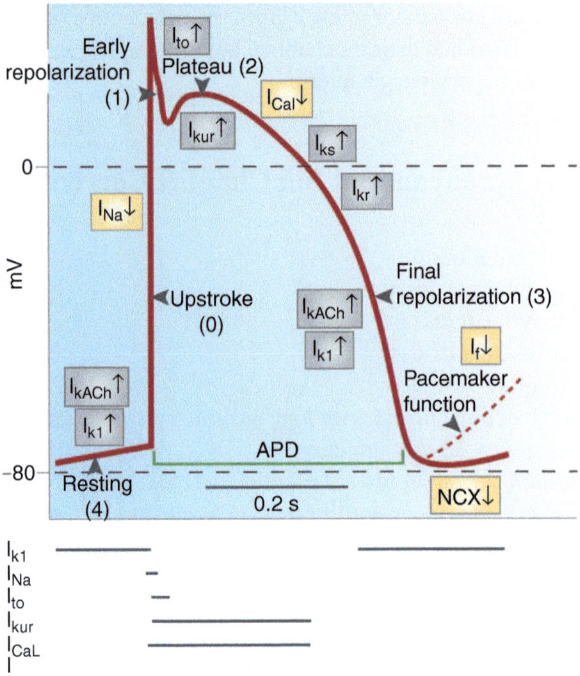

Fig. 9.1 Membrane currents that generate normal ventricular action potential upstroke (phase 0), overshoot and notch (phase1), slow phase of repolarization (plateau or phase 2), and fast phase of repolarization (phase 3 (and the resting potential (phase 4). *Broken line* shows the SA node in pacemaker potential. The inward currents, *I*Na, *I*Ca, and *I*f, are shown in *yellow boxes*; the electrogenic sodium-calcium exchanger (NCX) is also shown in *yellow* although it may generate inward or outward current. The outward currents I_{KAch}, I_{K1}, I_{to}, I_{Kur}, *I*Kr, and I_{Ks} are shown in *gray boxes* (Reproduced from Nattel and Carlsson [2], with permission)

9.2 Ion Channel Currents Modulating Ventricular Action Potential Duration

These currents include inward calcium currents (I_{Ca}), transient outward potassium currents I_{to} and I_{Kur} and delayed rectifier K^+currents I_{Kr} and IKs shown in Fig. 9.1. ICa^{2+} is involved with both of these categories in regulating ventricular APD. IKr is the rapidly activating outward rectifying potassium current and IKs the slowly activating outward rectifying potassium current.

The impact of Ito on phase 2 of action potential is through opening of Ca^{2+} channels thereby modulating action potential duration (APD). Left ventricular epicardial layers where repolarization normally starts have higher levels of Ito expression. The rate of Ito inactivation is variable and highly voltage-dependent. α-adrenergic stimulation reduces *I*to in human myocytes through PKA-dependent phosphorylation. Chronic α-adrenergic stimulation and anangiotensin II also reduces channel expression. In large mammals *I*to reduction shifts phase 2 plateau to more positive potentials increasing the activation of the delayed rectifier (K^+ currents IKr and IKs in Fig. 9.1) and promoting faster repolarization. *I*Ks is expressed in all cell types, but is reduced in midmyocardial myocytes. These cells have the longest action potential duration across the myocardial wall.

9.3 Inward Calcium Current

For the inward calcium currents (I_{Ca}) the labels are assigned based on their time-dependent properties. The label I_{CaL} signifies long-lasting and label T in I_{CaT} refers to transient. I_{CaT} channels are scarce or absent in mammalian ventricular myocytes. In atria, I_{CaT} current is carried through a different voltage-gated ionic channel and it may be associated with abnormal automaticity described later. The main focus here is on I_{CaL} in ventricular myocytes.

I_{CaL} activation occurs with a delay with respect of depolarization (which is brought about by inward I_{Na} current, phase 0 of the action potential) has reached a lower level of membrane potential. The activated state of I_{CaL} is long lasting. It is important for excitation-contraction coupling by triggering the release of intracellular Ca^{2+}. The balance of inward I_{CaL} current and K^+ efflux determines to a large extent the quasi-stationary equilibrium during phase 2 (the slow phase of repolarization generally called "plateau"). I_{CaL} is thus an important determinant of phase 2 duration and the onset of the fast phase of repolarization (phase 3) occurring at the inactivation of I_{CaL} as shown in Fig. 9.1. With inactivation of I_{CaL} the outward potassium current with its high concentrations gradient becomes a dominant force in transmembrane ionic balance and the fast phase of repolarization (phase 3) starts. I_{CaL} is thus an important determinant of APD. Neurotransmitters and calcium channel blockers have a strong influence on I_{CaL}.

9.4 Resting Potential and Inward Rectifiers

From other voltage-gated outward potassium currents, I_{K1} is the "inward rectifier". I_{K1} channels have a high conductance when the membranes are polarized to a high negative value and I_{Kr} is important for maintaining the resting potential (phase 4). The conductance of I_{K1} is reduced sharply when the membrane potential decreases to above – 40 mV at the onset of depolarization (phase 0).

9.5 Pacemaker Potential of the Sino-Atrial Node

Ion channels contributing to phase 4 depolarization include If, IK^+ activated during the preceding action potential, ICaL and ICaT, background Na^+ current and the sodium-calcium exchanger (NCX). If is activated when the membrane potential falls below –40 mV when repolarization is completed.

Ito has a fast component in human atria. The SA node action potential has a steep slope and short duration in phase 2. Phase 3 starts and ends early and the resting potential starts decreasing immediately (pacemaker potential. The slope of this resting potential decline is rate-dependent and the rate-dependence is more pronounced in women than in men.

IKur is highly expressed in SA node and other atrial myocytes and is the basis for the much shorter duration of the action potential in atria than in ventricles. Ligand-dependent gating with Ach-activated K^+ current is a part of the mechanism of the vagal control of the heart rate. Derailed control SA nodes pacemaking activity in AF was covered in Chap. 5.

9.6 Drugs Modulating Cardiac Ion Channels

Classification of antiarrhythmic mechanisms proposed in 1991 by a Working Group on Arrhythmias of the European Society of Cardiology [3] is shown in Table 9.1. The table shows the desired antiarrhythmic effect on the most likely vulnerable period and ion currents most likely to achieve the desired effect.

Drugs modulating cardiac ion channels are in the realm of extensive electrophysiological and pharmacological research [4]. This subject area is beyond the scope of the present monograph. The next few paragraphs merely point out the vast range of normal and abnormal conditions related to the multitude of cardiac ion channels and gene mutations.

9.6.1 Potassium Channels and Channel Blockers

KCNH2, the hERG-gene codes for a protein labeled Kv11.1, the alpha subunit of a potassium channel. The hERG potassium channels are essential for normal electrical activity in the heart. Inherited LQTS is associated with mutations in the hERG gene predisposing individuals to life-threatening arrhythmias. Arrhythmia can also be induced by a blockage of hERG channels by a large number of diverse cardioactive agents which has caused disappointing results for many preclinical drug safety studies.

The origin of the label 'Ether-à-go-go' denoting the hERG-gene is interesting. According to Wikipedia, The hERG gene is the human homolog of the Ether-a-go-go gene found in the Drosophila fly and named in the 1960s by William D. Kaplan. When flies with mutations in this gene are anaesthetized with ether, their legs start to shake, like the legs of the dancers at the then popular 'Whisky A Go-Go' nightclub in West Hollywood.

Arrhythmias related to abnormal repolarization are commonly caused by mutations in genes encoding K^+-channels. Mutations in hHERG-gene and in gene encoding KvLQT1 cause the majority of Romano-Ward syndromes, autosomal dominant LQTS. Quinidine, procainamide, and disopyramide are examples of drugs that

Table 9.1 Categorization of arrhythmogenic mechanisms, desired antiarrhythmic effect on the most likely vulnerable parameter and ionic currents most likely to achieve the desired antiarrhythmic effect

Mechanism of arrhythmia	Antiarrhythmic effect on vulnerable parameter	Ionic currents most likely to achieve desired effect
Enhanced normal automaticity	Decrease rate of phase 4 depolarization	Block I_f, $I_{Ca\text{-}T}$
		Activate $I_{K(Ach)}$
Abnormal automaticity	Increase (hyperpolarize) max diastolic potential or decrease rate of phase 4 depolarization in latent focus	Activate I_K; $I_{K(Ach)}$
		Block $I_{Ca\text{-}L}$; I_{Na}
Triggered activity induced by EAD	Shorten APD	Activate I_K
		Block $I_{Ca\text{-}L}$; I_{Na}
Triggered activity induced by DAD	Reduce calcium overload or suppress DAD	Block $I_{Ca\text{-}L}$
		Block $I_{Ca\text{-}L}$; I_{Na}
Na channel dependent reentry with primary impaired conduction (long excitatory gap)	Decrease excitability and conduction	Block I_{Na}
Na channel-dependent reentry with conduction encroaching on refractoriness (short excitatory gap)	Prolong effective refractory period	Block I_K
Ca channel-dependent reentry	Decrease excitability and conduction	Block $I_{Ca\text{-}L}$
Reflection	Decrease excitability	Block $I_{Ca\text{-}L}$; I_{Na}
Parasystole	Decrease rate of phase 4 depolarization in automatic (Purkinje) focus	Block I_f (if max neg diastolic potential hyperpolarized)

Source: Task Force of the Working Group on Arrhythmias of the European Society of Cardiology [3] (Copyright © 1991 American Heart Association. Reproduced with permission from Lippincott, Williams & Wilkins)

EAD early afterdepolarizations, *DAD* delayed afterdepolarizations, *APD* action potential duration

block K^+-channel prolonging QT and in some setups causing TdP. Antiarrhythmic drugs have lost their appeal because of serious side effects although they are important in the management of patients with recurrent AF. IKur channel is a new target for search of new drugs for AF after discovery of atrial-specific distribution of IKur.

9.6.2 Ca^{2+}: Channel

Verapamil and diltiazem are examples of class IV drugs blocking open and inactivated Ca^{2+}- channels. The sudden cardiac death syndrome combining ECG features of the Brugada syndrome including short QT associated with a loss of function of the L-type Ca2 α1- or β2b subunit of the channel has been described by Antzelevitch et al. [5].

9.6.3 *If: Channel*

This channel has been targeted in search for agents (ivabradine etc.) which slow down heart rate without negative inotropic effect or hypotension which is the disadvantage of β-blockers. These drugs have been found effective in management of patients with stable angina pectoris. Newer findings include mutations of hyperpolarization-activated cyclic nucleotide-gated potassium channel 4 or HCN4 associated with idiopathic sinus bradycardia and chronotrophic incompetence in one family [6] and severe bradycardia, QT prolongation, and torsade de pointes in another family [5]. *If* expression is upregulated in cardiac hypertrophy and congestive heart failure and may contribute to the arrhythmias observed in these disease conditions.

9.7 QT Interval

9.7.1 *QT Rate-Adjustment Formulas*

A variety of formulas with substantial differences in functional form have been introduced in ECG literature for QT adjustment for heart rate variation [7, 8]. QT rate sensitivity in women is higher than in men (the slope coefficient in linear regression of QT vs. RR interval is larger in women than in men) and the rate sensitivity decreases with age in both gender groups. The formulas by Bazett [9] and Fridericia [10] introduced in 1920 continue to be most commonly used for QT rate adjustment in clinical applications. Bazett's formula (QTcBz) leaves a large bias in rate-adjusted QT at high and low heart rates by overcorrecting at higher heart rates and undercorrecting at low heart rates. This increases the proportion of false negative QT prolongations at high heart rates and false positives at low heart rates. The bias with Fridericia's formula (QTcFr) is in opposite direction to that with QTcBz although the bias is smaller in magnitude. Both of these two formulas ignore the gender difference in QT rate sensitivity. Another problem with many QT rate adjustment formulas is that they may produce a satisfactory rate adjustment of the mean or median QT but do not properly adjust upper limits of QT distribution [8].

Newer formulas introduced labeled QTcLogLin and QTcMod in Table 9.2 may reduce the problems noted above [8]. This table provides a framework for categorization of QTc formulas as linear and inverse based on their generic form and QT prediction function. Rate-adjusted upper normal limits are strongly age- and gender-dependent.

9.7.2 *Optimal Choice of QT Rate-Adjustment Formula*

Prognostic data in previous chapters have shown that QT has a limited role among predictors of mortality and other cardiac events as summarized in Sect. 9.9 below.

Table 9.2 Categorization of QTc formulas as linear and inverse based on their generic forms and QT prediction functions

QTc formula label	QT prediction function	Generic form of QTc in terms of QT prediction function (QTpr)	Men		Women	
			C[a]	k[b]	C	k
	Linear[c]					
QTcRR	RR^k	QTc=QT– Cx(QTpr-1)	154	1	168	1
QTcHR	HR^k	QTc=QT+Cx(60-QTpr)	2.0	1	2.07	1
QTcLog Lin	RR^k	QTc=QT–Cx(QTpr-1)	398	0.37	409	0.38
	Inverse[d]					
[e]QRcBz	RR^k	QTc=QT/CxQTpr	1	0.5	1	0.5
[f]QTcFr	RR^k	QTc=QT/CxQTpr	1	0.33	1	0.33
[d]QTcLogInv	RR^k	QTc=QT/CxQTpr	1	0.37	1	0.38
[g]QTcMod	$1/(120+HR^k)$	QTc=QT/CxQTpr	180	1	180	1

Modified from Rautaharju et al. [26] with permission
RR RR interval, *HR* heart rate
[a]C = slope coefficient of QTc formula
[b]k = exponent of the QT predicton function
[c]In linear adjustment of QT, the adjustment term is added to QT as a linear proportion of the difference of the prediction function from the reference interval or HR (RR=1 or HR=60)
[d]In inverse adjustment QT is divided by the prediction function
[e]QTcBz = Bazett's formula
[f]QTcFr = Fridericia's formula
[g]QTcMod = Modular QTc prediction formula

Certain pragmatic considerations may help in the choice of the QT rate-adjustment formula in a given clinical set-up: (1) Experience shows that the achievement of a universally satisfactory formula for QT rate adjustment is an elusive goal; (2) First of all, the use of QTcBz should be avoided; (3) Formulas with a separate adjustment for women and men are preferable; (4) Otherwise formulas which within physiological range of heart rates produce reasonably stable mean and upper limits for rate-adjusted QT work quite well for practical clinical applications; (5) Additional correction may be necessary for heart rates above 100/min or below 50/min; (6) Individual rate-adjustment with QT values measured over a wider range of heart rates from ambulatory ECGs may enhance the accuracy of QT rate adjustment. However, ambulatory ECGs are acquired in less standardized conditions than most of the routine 12-lead ECGs and induce additional dynamic variability from sources other than hear rate and autonomic balance; (7) In a clinical setup, QTc by any formula (excluding Bazett) exceeding 170 ms clearly indicates abnormal QT prolongation (if measurement is verified).

The fact that QT has its limitations does not diminish the importance of extra care in the choice of QT rate-adjustment procedures in evaluation of the safety of cardioactive drugs and other agents. In these applications, ECG measures of altered ST-T waveform and altered spatial direction of repolarization should be taken into consideration as information supplementary to QT. Separate measures are needed relating to the slow and fast phase of repolarization although identification of the demarcation point between them may at times have procedural problems.

Conceptually more important in terms of adverse outcomes are ECG measures of deviant spatial direction of regional LV lateral wall repolarization, Θ(Rp|Tp), and global measure of end of repolarization, TpTe interval.

9.7.3 Gender Differences in QT

Sex differences in rate-adjusted QT were traditionally thought to be due to QT prolongation in women making women more vulnerable to QT prolonging effects of certain drugs and cardioactive agents. However, a Canadian study [11] found that gender difference in QT is due QT shortening in adolescent boys and that QT remains shorter in men than in women through adulthood.

A recent report by Rautaharju et al. [8] evaluated sex differences in age-evolution of the rate-adjusted QT by in a study group of 45,952 persons aged 5–89 years (54 % women) excluding conditions with possible disease-associated ECG changes. A new QTcMod was derived in the study for QT rate adjustment (QTcMod = QT*(HR + 120)/188). Figure 9.2 highlights the gender differences in QT evolution in that large study group showing the QTc decrease in males during adolescence with no change in females. At age 20–24 years QTc was 14 ms longer in women than in men in spite of 6 ms longer QRS duration in men. After age 20 years QTc increased linearly through adulthood in both sex groups, with a steeper increase in men causing a gradual decrease in the sex difference. The results were closely similar with QT rate-adjustment using

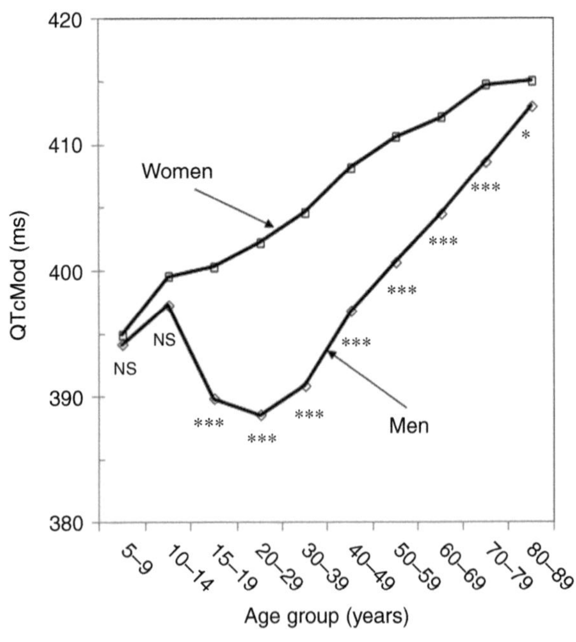

Fig. 9.2 Mean values of rate-adjusted QT by the QTcMod formula in men and women by age. QTc decreases in adolescent boys with no decrease in adolescent girls, and there is a gradual nearly linear increase with age in both sex groups of adults. *** signifies P<0.001, * P<0.05 and NS nonsignificant for *t*-test for sex differences between men and women (From Rautaharju et al. [8])

a gender-specific QTcLogLin formula (QTcLogLin = QT + 409x(1-RR$^{0.39}$) for women and QTcLogLin = QT + 387x(1-RR$^{0.37}$) for men).

The observed shorter QTcMod in men than in women is unexpected on two accounts: the rate-adjusted QT is commonly thought to be due to QT prolongation in women and secondly because QRS duration is longer in men than in women reflecting higher left ventricular mass. More recent studies have demonstrated that the shorter rate-adjusted QT in men than in women is associated with an earlier start and earlier end of left ventricular (LV) epicardial repolarization [12, 13]. However, QRS duration still contributes to QT prolongation during the terminal repolarization which is predominantly concordant with respect to depolarization sequence.

9.7.4 The Mechanism of Gender Differences Rate-Adjusted QT

Although Fig. 9.1 is very informative about ion currents involved in modifying APD, it does not explain gender differences in action potential waveforms and APD. Figure 9.3 was constructed as a schematic for possible mechanisms to account for these gender differences. Labels for ion channel currents at different action potential phases accounting for gender differences are shown with upward arrows indicating outward currents and downward arrows inward currents. Increased I_{to} causes ST segment dome shift to higher potential level in males (A) reduces APD, enhances activation of the delayed rectifiers ($I_{Ks,}I_{Kr}$) and promotes faster repolarization. Furthermore, phase 2 descent is faster and phase 3 repolarization is slower in males than in females (B). According to the repolarization model this accounts for the asymmetric ST-T waveform in males with upsloping U-shaped ST segment and tall T wave.

APepi and APendo differences in women at action potential (AP) phase 2 are minimal and consequently STJ-point elevation is absent and ST segment flat in women. Kir2.3 levels in females at epicardium have been found lower than at endocardium [14]. Kir2.3 is a channel subunit which mediates cardiac inward rectifier I_{K1}. The expected result according to the repolarization model: RTepi is prolonged more than RTendo, QTpa prolongs and crossmural dispersion of the end of repolarization (TpTxd interval) increases. QT increases if TpTe remains unchanged or increases (by reduced IK1 prolonging phase 3 also at basal regions normally repolarising last). A more pronounced APD prolongation in females may account for the more pronounced arrhythmogenic effect in Brugada and LQTSin women than in men.

The schematic in Fig. 9.4 illustrates the dependence of normal female ST-T waveform on the waveform of APepi. These two functions have a common link in their convexity. ST-T segment convexity (Co) evaluated at time point of Tonset is defined by the repolarization model positive because the ST-T segment is ‘U-shaped’ and lies below the line drawn from the J-Point to the peak of the T wave. The convexity of AP_{epi} is negative because it is ‘dome-shaped’ and lies above the line drawn from the beginning of phase 2 to the end of phase 3.

Gender differences in ST-T waveforms are highlighted in Fig. 9.5. The convexity of the ST-T wave in J-Tpeak interval is reduced in males compared to females. This

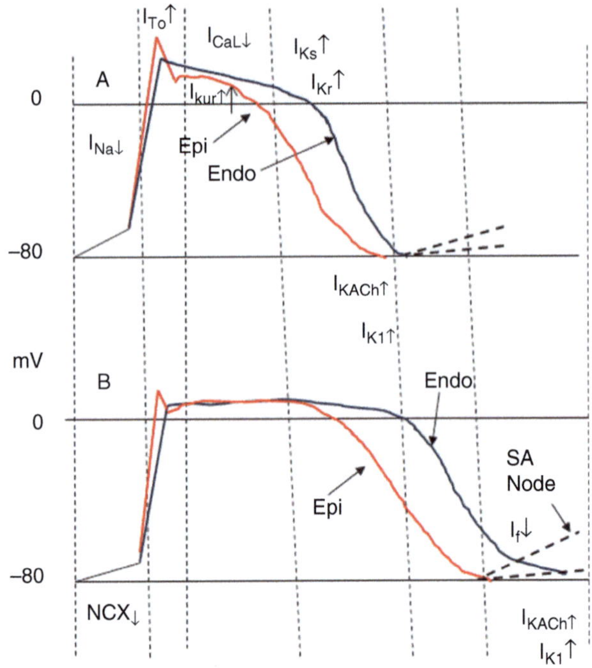

Fig. 9.3 A schematic for epicardial (Epi, *red curves*) and endocardial (Endo, *blue curves*) action potential waveforms in males (*A*, *top curves*) and females (*B*, *bottom curves*). Labels for ion channel currents at different action potential phases accounting for gender differences are shown with *upward arrows* indicating outward currents and *downward arrows* inward currents. ST segment dome shift to higher potential level in males reduces APD, enhances activation of the delayed rectifiers ($I_{Ks,}I_{Kr}$) and promotes faster repolarization. Resting membrane potential is determines by I_{KAcH} and I_{K1}. I_f ion current modifies the slope of phase 4 resting potential of SA node pacemaker potential (*broken lines*). Compared to males the slope in females has increased rate-dependence

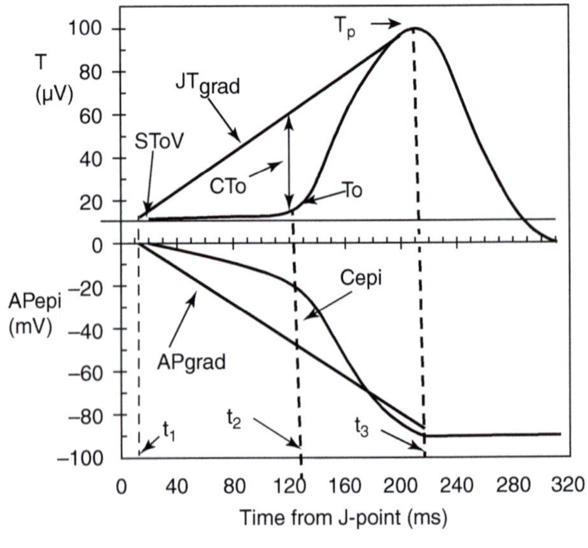

Fig. 9.4 A schematic illustrating the dependence of the convexity of the female ST segment (CTo) on the convexity of epicardial action potential (Cepi). The convexity of both functions is evaluated at time point of the onset of the T wave (To) which in epicardial action potential (APepi) coincides with the start of the fast phase or repolarization (phase 3). The special feature of female ST-T curve is the relatively 'flat' ST segment followed by a fast rising curve in the ascending limb of the T wave after To

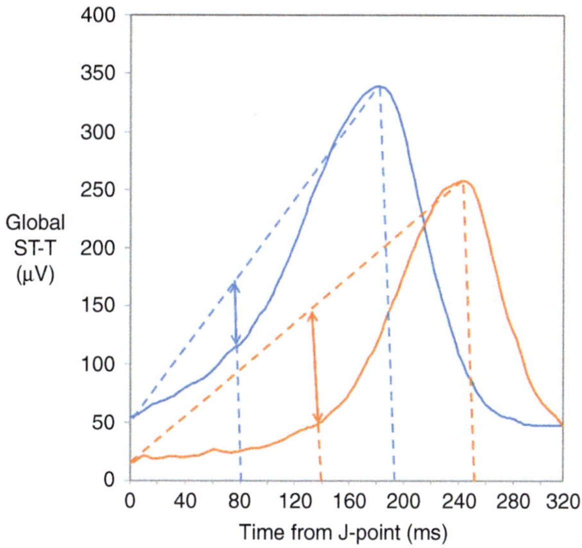

Fig. 9.5 Characteristic waveforms of the global ST-T waves distinguishing female (*orange curve*) from male (*blue*) patterns. The convexity of the female ST segment from the J-point to the peak of T (Tp) is high. The convexity of the ST-T curve in men is lower, with an earlier start and end of repolarization of the left ventricular lateral wall and shorter JTp interval tin men than han in women. QTe interval is longer in women than in men although TpTe interval representing global dispersion of repolarization is longer in men than in women

is due to earlier start and earlier completion of repolarization of the left ventricular lateral wall. The rate-adjusted QT is longer in women than in men although TpTe interval is longer in men than in women.

9.7.4.1 The Role of Testosterone

QT intervals in the highest and lowest quartiles of total and free testosterone levels were compared by Zhang et al. in men enrolled in the Third National Health and Nutrition Examination Survey and men and postmenopausal women enrolled in the Multi-Ethnic Study of Atherosclerosis (MESA) [15]. Significant differences were observed in the multivariable-adjusted QT intervals between the highest and lowest quartiles of testosterone in men but not in women. The authors concluded that testosterone may account for the shorter QT intervals in men than in women.

Bidoggia et al. in a small clinical study of 106 patients found that QT was prolonged in castrated men compared with noncastrated men and that women with hyperandrogenism had shorter QT-interval durations than the control [16]. Therapeutic testosterone administration was associated with significant QT-interval shortening in a small clinical study on hypogonadic men by Charbit et al. [17]. Testosterone modulates the main depolarizing current (L-typeCa^{2+}) at phase 2 of ventricular AP and a primary repolarizing current (I_{Ks}) during phase 3, shortening APD and QT. Taken together, these studies support the assertion that testosterone-associated altered dynamics of cardiac ion channels account for the shorter rate-adjusted QT in men. The sex difference might be even greater if it weren't for longer QRS durations in men than in women.

9.8 ST-T Waveforms: The Mechanism for Gender Differences

This section contains a brief summary of the main factors accounting for gender differences in ST-T waveforms.

9.8.1 Male ST-T Waveform Pattern

Increased transient outward potassium current (I_{to}) shifts ST segment dome to higher potential level in males, reduces APD, enhances activation of the delayed rectifiers ($I_{Ks,}I_{Kr}$) and promotes faster repolarization at action potential phase 2 and phase 3 thus generating the asymmetric T waveform with upsloping 'U-shaped' ST segment and tall T wave.

9.8.2 Female ST-T Waveform Pattern

Epicardial and endocardial action potential differences in women at phase 2 are minimal, STJ-point elevation amplitude is low (mostly below 50 μV) and ST segment is flat. Potassium channel subunit Kir2.3 levels in females at epicardium have been found to be lower than at endocardium. Kir2.3 mediates cardiac inward rectifier I_{K1}. The expected result of lower Kir2.3 level is that RTepi is prolonged more than RTendo, QTpa prolongs and crossmural dispersion of the end of repolarization (TpTxd interval) increases and also QT increases if TpTe remains unchanged or increases (by reduced I_{K1} prolonging phase 3 at basal regions normally repolarising last).

9.8.3 Common Mechanism for Gender Differences in ST Elevation and QTinterval

Gender differences in the evolution of ST elevation are most prominent in anterior chest lead V2 as reported by Ezaki et al. [18]. Figure 9.6a, b show the mean J-point elevation values by age from the report of Ezaki et al. displayed side-by-side with QTcMod values adjusted for age in addition to heart rate. Figure 9.6a, b show that the time course of the shortening of QT in adolescence males parallels the time course of the increase of STJ amplitude. This suggests that gender differences arising in adolescence in age-evolution of QT and ST have some neurohormonal factor, most likely testosterone, as a common mechanism [19]. This interesting postulate needs further research.

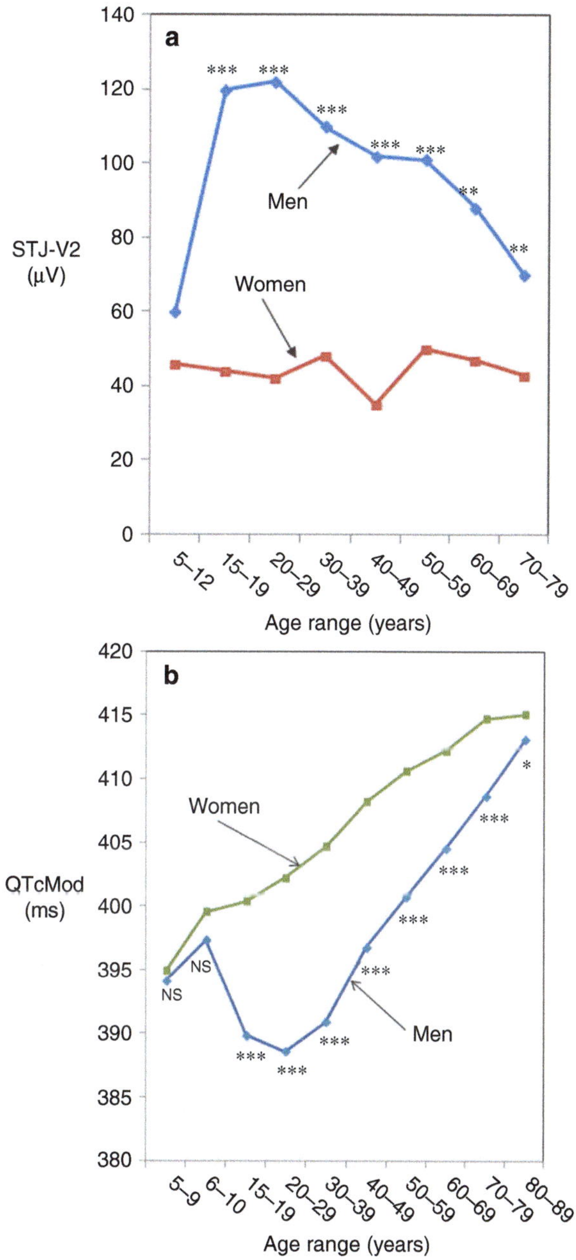

Fig. 9.6 (**a**, **b**) J-point elevation (**a**) by age displayed side-by-side with QTcMod (**b**). The comparison of these figures suggests that gender differences arising in adolescence inST elevation and QT are caused by a common neurohormonal mechanism, most likely by testosterone. ***signifies P<0.001, **P<0.01, *P<0.05 and NS non-significant gender difference (**a** Is from Fig. 2A, [18], with permission, **b** is from Rautaharju et al. [8])

9.8.4 QRS/T Angle in Acute Coronary Syndrome

Several studies have emphasized the importance of various QRS/T angles as predictors of adverse cardiac events. QRS/T angle has also been associated with mortality risk in the general clinical population [20] and in acute coronary syndrome (ACS) [21, 22].

The postulated mechanism for QRS/T angle widening in ACS involves the following chain of events: Ischemia most commonly in anterior wall induces APD shortening in ischemic subepicardial layers and changes the direction of lateral wall repolarization and Tp|Tref angle widens. The ion channel mechanisms are thought to be associated with the ATP-sensitive K_ channel, also termed the ADP-activated K_ channel, which is a ligand-gated channel distributed abundantly in all regions of the heart [1]. The open probability of this channel is proportional to the [ADP]/[ATP] ratio. The shape of the action potential depends on the metabolic state of the cell. Energy depletion during ischemia increases the [ADP]/[ATP] ratio, activates *I*K ATP, and abbreviates the action potential. Contractile force is reduced when APD shortens which may be cardioprotective. The channel is important also in ischemic preconditioning.

9.9 Independent Predictors of Adverse Cardiac Events

Sex differences in ion channel currents modulating action potential durations are not only of interest from the perspective of electrophysiological mechanisms to elucidate their mechanism but they have practical clinical implications briefly summarized here from the data in previous chapters.

9.9.1 Independent Predictors for Heart Failure

Increased QRS nondipolar voltage and two angular variables, Θ(R|STT) and Θ(Tp|Tref) in women were independent predictors of HF, with an approximately 60 % increased risk for all (Chap. 5, Table 5.2). Wide Θ(Tp|Tref) was an independent predictor of HF also in men, but otherwise the predictors in men differed from those in women. In men prolonged RTepi and prolonged TpTe interval and T wave complexity were independent predictors of incident HF, with 62 % increased risk for RTepi and approximately 30 % increased risk for TpTe interval and T wave complexity. TpTe interval reflects global dispersion of the end of repolarization and T wave complexity the roundness of T wave vector loop.

I_{to} current is reduced in human heart failure and in this condition it is associated with a prolongation of the action potential duration [1]. Ito may thus be involved in the mechanisms for HF.

The synergistic actions of AF and HF reinforcing the occurrence of each others was covered in Chap. 5. Heart rate alone commonly comes up as a predictor of diverse adverse outcomes. In the MESA study elevated resting heart rate related to development of regional and global LV dysfunction was associated with increased risk for incident HF in asymptomatic participants [23]. The development of regional and global LV dysfunction was independent of subclinical atherosclerosis and coronary heart disease.

9.9.2 *Independent Predictors for Sudden Cardiac Death*

QT prolongation has been associated with SCD in several studies (Table 6.1 in Chap. 6). ECG-estimate of left ventricular mass (LVMI) was also a predictor for SCD. Of particular interest is the role of Θ(Tp|Tref) as the strongest independent predictor of SCD in CVD-free women with 3.55-fold increased risk and in CVD-free men with a 1.91-fold increased risk (Table 6.2 in Chap. 6). The remaining independent predictors were different in women from those in men: Θ(Rm|Tm) and TV1 amplitude in women, and in men Θ(Tinit|Tterm) and QTea. A noteworthy observation is the 3.55-fold increased risk for SCD for Θ(Tp|Tref) in women. QTea was an independent predictor in men but not in women.

9.9.3 *Independent Predictors for CHD Death*

In postmenopausal women $\Theta(T_{p|}T_{ref})$ >42° and TaVR amplitude less negative than −100 μV were the strongest independent predictors in women with and without CVD with an over twofold increased risk for both(Table 4.3, Chap. 4).

Comparing sex differences in independent predictors of CHD death in CVD-free women and men in the ARIC study, Θ(Rm|Tm) and TV1 amplitude were the strongest predictors in women, with over twofold increased risk for both (Table 4.7, Chap. 4). In men the strongest independent predictors were Θ(Rm|Tm) and TaVR amplitude, with 40 % increased risk for Θ(Rm|Tm) and 54 % increased risk for TaVR. QT prolongation was an independent predictor in men (48 % increased risk) but not in women.

9.10 ST Deviations as CVD Death Predictors in the Copenhagen Heart Study

In Copenhagen Heart Study ST-depressions in nearly all chest leads were associated with a dose-responsive increased risk of CVD [24]. In young men STelevations in V2–V3 were associated with a decreased risk of CVD. In women and in older men ST-elevations were associated with increased risk of CVD in women and with regard to lead V1 also in men. Consistent with findings associated with ECG-LVH in other studies covered in Chap. 7, the highest risk was found for ECG-LVH associated with LVH strain pattern.

9.11 Upper Normal Limits for STJ Elevation in V1 and V2 in the Netherlands Study

Rijnbeek et al. in their extensive well-documented study from four predominantly white populations in the Netherlands established upper normal limits for a comprehensive set of ECG variables in men and women aged from 16 to 90 years, including STJ elevation in chest leads V1 and V2 in age groups younger than 40 years [25]. Figure 9.7 derived from the Supplementary Table 8 of that report shows in adult women 150 μV can be suggested as a practical upper normal limit for ST elevation. In younger adult men ST elevation in V2 reflects normal cardiac adaptation to increased physical activity level rather than as a marker of increased risk. In V1, on the other hand, ST elevation in both men and women was associated with increased risk for CVD in Copenhagen heart study. Therefore, 100 μV is suggested as a practical upper limit for STJ elevation in V1 in white adult women, 120 μV in white younger men and 110 μV in white older men (Fig. 9.8). In North-American populations racial differences in ST amplitudes in women (Figs. B1 and B2) and the substantially higher STJ amplitudes in African-American men than in women (Figs. C8 and C9) are an important consideration particularly in age groups older than 40 years when the prevalence and incidence of adverse CVD events start increasing.

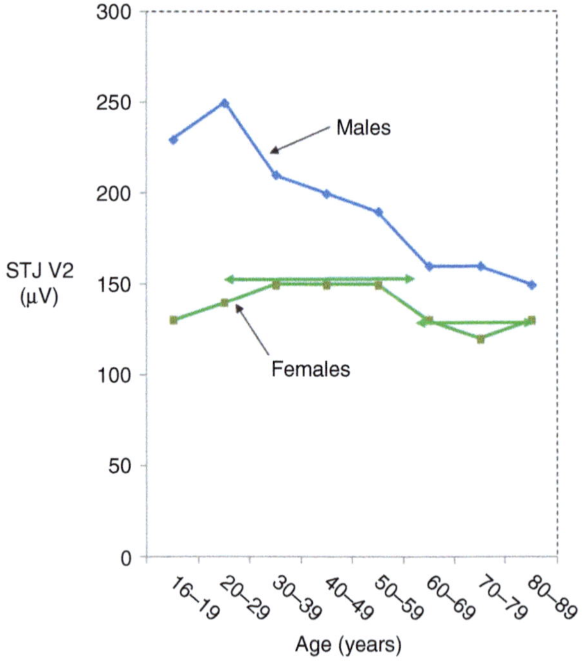

Fig. 9.7 ST J-point amplitudes in adolescent and adult females and males in V2. In adult women 150 μV (*double arrow*) is suggested as the upper normal limit for ST elevation. In younger adult men ST elevation in V2 reflects normal cardiac adaptation to increased physical activity level particularly in athletes. The upper normal limits (98th percentiles) decrease in older women and particularly in older men (Adapted from Supplementary Table 8 in Rijnbeek et al. [25])

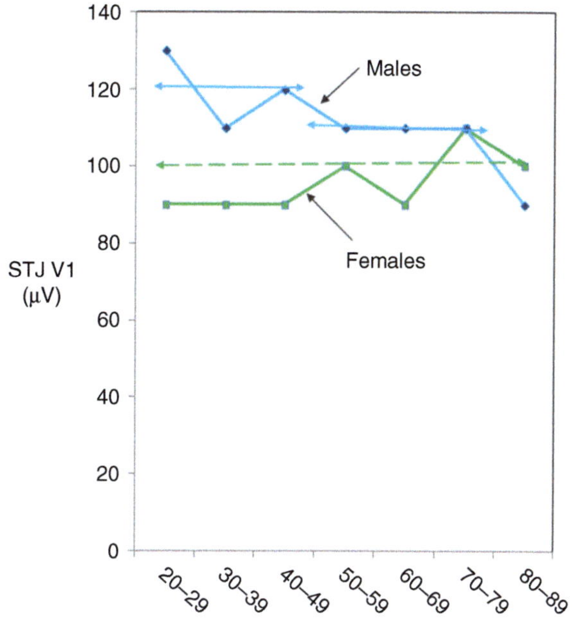

Fig. 9.8 ST J-point amplitudes in adolescent and adult females and males in V1. The horizontal dashed double arrow represents the suggested practical upper normal limit for adult women. The solid double arrows indicate suggested upper normal limits in younger and older men (120 and 110 μV, respectively) (Adapted from Supplementary Table 8 in Rijnbeek et al. [25])

9.12 Age-Dependence of QT Adjusted for Heart Rate by QTcMod Formula

Dependence on age of the QT interval adjusted for heart rate (HR) by QTcMod formula (QTcMod = QT*(120 + HR)/180 for men and women) was documented by Rautaharju et al. in a large North-American clinically normal population [8]. Figure 9.9a (on the left) reproduced from Fig. 9.4 of that report shows a strong trend with age in QTcMod in adults. Figure 9.9b shows that a residual age-trend remains in QTcMod even after removal of linear age trend both in women and men. This residual age trend reflects most likely QT increase with gradually evolving subclinical CHD.

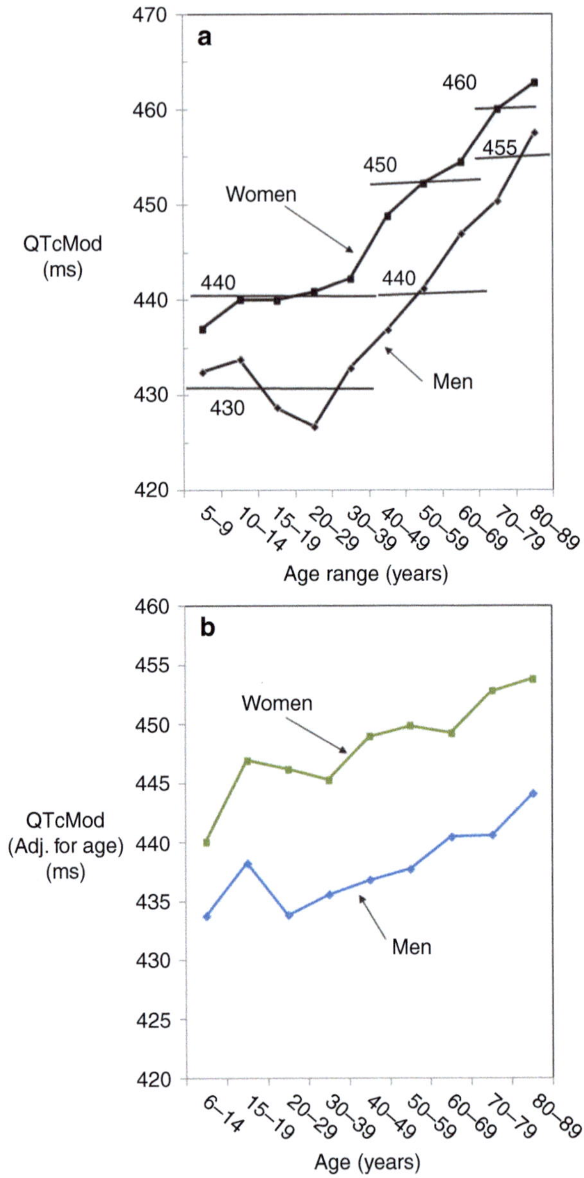

Fig. 9.9 (**a**, **b**) Age trend in QT adjusted for heart rate by the QTcMod formula (*on the left*) and residual age trend remaining in QTcMod after removal of linear age trend (*on the right*). This residual age trend in (**b**) reflects most likely QT increase with gradually evolving subclinical CHD (Reproduced from Fig. 4, Rautaharju et al. [8], with permission)

References

1. Grant AO. Cardiac ion channels. Circ Arrhythm Electrophysiol. 2009;2:185–94.
2. Nattel S, Carlsson L. Innovative approaches to anti-arrhythmic drug therapy. Nat Rev Drug Discov. 2006;5:1034–49.
3. A new approach to the classification of antiarrhythmic drugs based on their actions on arrhythmogenic mechanisms. Task Force of the Working Group on Arrhythmias of the European Society of Cardiology. The Sicilian gambit. Circulation. 1991;84:1831–51.
4. Kurokawa J, Kodama M, Furukawa T, Clancy EE. Sex and gender aspects in antiarrhythmic therapy. In: Regitz-Zagrosek V, editor. Sex and gender differences in pharmacology. London: Springer. 2012; p. 237–64.
5. Antzelevitch C, Pollevick GD, Cordeiro JM, Casis O, Sanguinetti MC, Aizawa Y, Guerchicoff A, Pfeiffer R, Oliva A, Wollnik B, Gelber P, Bonaros Jr EP, Burashnikov E, Wu Y, Sargent JD, Schickel S, Oberheiden R, Bhatia A, Hsu L-F, Haïssaguerre M, Schimpf R, Borggrefe M, Wolpert C. Loss-of-function mutations in the cardiac calcium channel underlie a new clinical entity characterized by ST-segment elevation, short QT intervals, and sudden cardiac death. Circulation. 2007;115:442–9.
6. Herrmann S, Hofmann F, Stieber J, Ludwig A. HCN channels in the heart: lessons from mouse mutants. Br J Pharmacol. 2012;166:501–9.
7. Malik M. Problems of HR correction in assessment of drug-induced QT interval prolongation. J Cardiovasc Electrophysiol. 2001;12:411–20.
8. Rautaharju PM, Mason JW, Akiyama T. New age- and sex-specific criteria for QT prolongation based on rate correction formulas that minimize bias at the upper normal limits. Int J Cardiol. 2014;174(3):535–40. Erratum in: Internat J Cardiol 2014;174(x):xxx.
9. Bazett H. An analysis of the time-relations of electrocardiograms. Heart. 1920;7:353–70.
10. Fridericia LS. Die Systolendauer im electrokardiogram bei normalen Menschen and bei Herzkranken. Acta Med Scand. 1920;53:469.
11. Rautaharju PM, Zhou SH, Wong S, Calhoun HP, Berenson GS, Prineas R, Davignon A. Sex differences in the evolution of the electrocardiographic QT interval with age. Can J Cardiol. 1992;8:690–5.
12. Rautaharju PM, Zhou SH, Gregg RE, Startt-Selvester RH. Electrocardiographic estimates of action potential durations and transmural repolarization time gradients in healthy subjects and in acute coronary syndrome patients–profound differences by sex and by presence vs absence of diagnostic ST elevation. J Electrocardiol. 2011;44:309–19.
13. Rautaharju PM, Gregg RE, Zhou SH, Startt-Selvester RH. Electrocardiographic estimates of regional action potential durations and repolarization time subintervals reveal ischemia-induced abnormalities in acute coronary syndrome not evident from global QT. J Electrocardiol. 2011;44:718–24.
14. Gaborit N, Varro A, Le Bouter S, Escande D, Nattel S, Demolombe S. Gender-related differences in ion-channel and transporter subunit expression in non-diseased human hearts. J Mol Cell Cardiol. 2010;49:639–46.
15. Zhang Y, Ouyang P, Post WS, Dalal D, Vaidya D, Blasco-Colmenares E, Soliman EZ, Tomaselli GF, Guallar E. Sex-steroid hormones and electrocardiographic QT-interval duration: findings from the third National Health and Nutrition Examination Survey and the Multi-Ethnic Study of Atherosclerosis. Am J Epidemiol. 2011;174:403–11.
16. Bidoggia H, Maciel JP, Capalozza N, Mosca S, Blaksley EJ, Valverde E, Bertran G, Arini P, Biagetti MO, Quinteiro RA. Sex differences on the electrocardiographic pattern of cardiac repolarization: possible role of testosterone. Am Heart J. 2000;140:678–83.
17. Charbit B, Christin-Maître S, Démolis JL, Soustre E, Young J, Funck-Brentano C. Effects of testosterone on ventricular repolarization in hypogonadic men. Am J Cardiol. 2009;103:887–90.

18. Ezaki K, Nakagawa M, Taniguchi Y, Nagano Y, Teshima Y, Yufu K, Takahashi N, Nomura T, Satoh F, Mimata H, Saikawa T. Gender differences in the ST segment-effect of androgen-deprivation therapy and possible role of testosterone. Circ J. 2010;74:2448–1454.
19. Rautaharju PM, Zhang ZM, Haisty Jr WK, Gregg RE, Warren J, Horaĉek MB, Kucharska-Newton AM, Rosamond W, Soliman EZ. Race- and sex-associated differences in rate-adjusted QT, QTpeak, ST elevation and other regional measures of repolarization: the Atherosclerosis Risk in Communities (ARIC) study. J Electrocardiol. 2014;47:342–50.
20. Yamazaki T, Froelicher VF, Myers J, Chun S, Wang P. Spatial QRS-T angle predicts cardiac death in a clinical population. Heart Rhythm. 2005;2:73–8.
21. Lown MT, Munyombwe T, Harrison W, West RM, Phil D, Hall AS, Gale CP, Evaluation of Methods and Management of Acute Coronary Events (EMMACE) Investigators. Association of frontal QRS-T angle–age risk score on admission electrocardiogram with mortality in patients admitted with an acute coronary syndrome. Am J Cardiol. 2012;109:307–13.
22. Rautaharju PM, Zhou SH, Gregg RE, Startt-Selvester RH. Heart rate, gender differences, and presence versus absence of diagnostic ST elevation as determinants of spatial QRS|T angle widening in acute coronary syndrome. Am J Cardiol. 2011;107:1744–50.
23. Opdahl A, Ambale Venkatesh B, Fernandes VR, Wu CO, Nasir K, Choi EY, Almeida AL, Rosen B, Carvalho B, Edvardsen T, Bluemke DA, Lima JA. Resting heart rate as predictor for left ventricular dysfunction and heart failure: MESA (Multi-Ethnic Study of Atherosclerosis). J Am Coll Cardiol. 2014;63:1182–9.
24. Rasmussen PV, Nielsen JB, Pietersen A, Graff C, Lind B, Struijk JJ, Olesen MS, Haunsø S, Køber L, Svendsen JH, Holst AG. Electrocardiographic precordial ST-segment deviations and the risk of cardiovascular death: results from the Copenhagen ECG Study. J Am Heart Assoc. 2014;3(3):e000549. doi:10.1161/JAHA.113.000549.
25. Rijnbeek PR, van Herpen G, Bots ML, Man S, Verweij N, Hofman A, Hillege H, Numans ME, Swenne CA, Witteman JCM, Kors JA. Normal values of the electrocardiogram for ages 16–90 years. J Electrocardiol. 2014;47:914–21.
26. Rautaharju PM, et al. New age- and sex-specific criteria for QT prolongation based on rate correction formulas that minimize bias at the upper normal limits. Int J Cardiol. 2014; 174:535–40.

Appendix A

Table A1 Heart rate, PR interval, QRS duration and unadjusted QT interval in white and African-American women aged 40–59 years

Variable	Statistic	White (n = 2,252)	African-American (n = 778)
Heart rate (cpm)	Mean; SD	68; 9.6	68; 10.3
	2→98 %	60→90	50→92
PR interval (ms)	Mean; SD	155; 21.9	166; 23.9
	2→98 %	124→202	124→216
QRS duration (ms)	Mean; SD	87; 7.8	86; 8.2
	2→98 %	80→106	70→104
QT interval (ms)	Mean; SD	398; 26.4	398; 29.4
	2→98 %	376→456	344→461

Modified from Rautaharju P, Rautaharju F. *Investigative electrocardiography in epidemiological studies and clinical trials*. London: Springer; 2007. p 1–289

P.M. Rautaharju, *The Female Electrocardiogram: Special Repolarization Features, Gender Differences, and the Risk of Adverse Cardiac Events*,
DOI 10.1007/978-3-319-15293-6

Table A2 P wave amplitudes and durations in white and African-American women aged 40–59 years, including the lower to upper ('→') second and fifth percentile normal limits for variables used in ECG criteria for right and left atrial enlargement

Variable	Statistic	White (N=2,252)	African-American (N=778)
PII duration (ms)	% Observed[a]	100	100
	Mean; SD	103; 11.8	108; 12.2
	2→98 %	80→126	86→132
PII amplitude >0 μV	% Observed	100	99
	Mean; SD	118; 40.3	122; 41.5
	2→98 %	43→205	43→209
PV1 duration (ms)	% Observed	99	99
	Mean; SD	59; 25.9	64; 26.8
	2→98 %	28→118	30→124
PV1 amplitude >0 μV	% Observed	95	98
	Mean; SD	45; 19.2	51; 20.5
	2→98 %	14→87	14→101
PPV1 duration (ms)	% Observed	55	60
	Mean; SD	60; 11.8	63; 12.2
	2→98 %	29→82	39→87
PPV1 amplitude <0 μV	% Observed	60	60
	Mean; SD	−41; 17.3	−41; 17.3
	2→98 %	−97→−24	−97→−24

Modified from Rautaharju P, Rautaharju F. *Investigative electrocardiography in epidemiological studies and clinical trials*. London: Springer; 2007. p 1–289

[a]Percentage women with corresponding P wave component

Table A3 Limb lead Q wave duration statistics including small Q waves[a] in white and African-American women aged 40–59 years

Lead/measurement	Statistic	White (N=2,252)	African-American (N=778)
aVL Q duration (ms)	% Obs[b]	31	46
	Mean; SD	20; 4.1	19; 3.8
	2→98 %	13→29	12→27
I Q duration (ms)	% Obs	44	45
	Mean; SD	18; 3.3	17; 3.4
	2→98 %	12→26	11→24
II Q duration (ms)	% Obs	49	26
	Mean; SD	18; 3.7	17; 3.9
	2→98 %	11→26	10→27
aVF Q duration (ms)	% Obs	46	25
	Mean; SD	20; 4.8	19; 4.9
	2→98 %	12→31	11→30
III Q duration (ms)	% Obs	44	27
	Mean; SD	24; 8.3	26; 8.9
	2→98 %	12→44	12→45

Modified from Rautaharju P, Rautaharju F. *Investigative electrocardiography in epidemiological studies and clinical trials*. London: Springer; 2007. p 1–289

[a]Q amplitude ≥25 μV and R amplitude ≥100 μV

[b]Percent women with small Q waves excluding QS

Table A4 Chest lead V4–V6 Q wave duration statistics for smaller and larger Q waves[a] in white and African-American women aged 40–59 years

Variable	Statistic	White (N=2,252)	African-American (N=778)
Small Q waves			
V5 Q duration (ms)	% Observed	41	32
	Mean; SD	17; 3.4	16; 3.6
	2→98 %	11→25	11→24
V6 Q duration (ms)	% Observed	60	45
	Mean; SD	18; 3.4	17; 3.4
	2→98 %	12→26	17→25
Larger Q waves			
V5 Q duration (ms)	% Observed	8	7
	Mean; SD	21; 2.8	20; 2.9
	2→98 %	16→28	15→25
V6 Q duration (ms)	% Observed	12	10
	Mean; SD	22; 2.7	21; 3.1
	2→98 %	17→28	16→27

Modified from Rautaharju P, Rautaharju F. *Investigative electrocardiography in epidemiological studies and clinical trials*. London: Springer; 2007. p 1–289

[a]Smaller Q Waves: Q amplitude 25–99 μV and R amplitude ≥100 μV; Larger Q waves: Q amplitude ≥100 μV and R amplitude ≥100 μV

Table A5 Limb lead R wave amplitudes in white and African-American women aged 40–59 years

Lead	Statistic	White (N=2,252)	African-American (N=778)
aVL amplitude (μV)	% Observed	82	92
	Mean; SD	426; 252.3	574; 310.4
	2→98 %	111→1,065	123→1,313
I amplitude (μV)	% Observed	100	100
	Mean; SD	701; 289.3	924; 326.8
	2→98 %	219→1,411	339→1,625
-aVR amplitude (μV)	% Observed	100	100
(Inverted aVR)	Mean; SD	444; 166.9	559; 184.3
	2→98 %	166→842	225→961
II amplitude (μV)	% Observed	100	99
	Mean; SD	881; 305.0	973; 349.7
	2→98 %	146→1,360	291→1,832
aVF amplitude (μV)	% Observed	94	93
	Mean; SD	604; 305.5	597; 322.8
	2→98 %	131→1,331	126→1,431
III amplitude (μV)	% Observed	74	71
	Mean; SD	470; 294.6	393; 288.6
	2→98 %	107→1,186	112→1,000

Modified from Rautaharju P, Rautaharju F. *Investigative electrocardiography in epidemiological studies and clinical trials*. London: Springer; 2007. p 1–289

Table A6 Chest lead R wave amplitudes in white and African-American women aged 40–59 years

Variable	Statistic	White (N=2,252)	African-American (N=778)
V1 amplitude[a] (μV)	% Observed	96	96
	Mean; SD	193; 120.2	199; 124.4
	2→98 %	39→502	34→522
V2 amplitude[a] (μV)	% Observed	100	99
	Mean; SD	452; 261.9	482; 298.7
	2→98 %	87→1,147	87→1,206
V3 amplitude (μV)	% Observed	99	99
	Mean; SD	792; 403.2	886; 454.1
	2→98 %	175→1,743	200→1,937
V4 amplitude (μV)	% Observed	100	100
	Mean; SD	1,198; 418.8	1,362; 479.2
	2→98 %	415→2,172	466→2,519
V5 amplitude (μV)	% Observed	100	100
	Mean; SD	1,210; 360.2	1,408; 421.6
	2→98 %	532→2,041	677→2,408
V6 amplitude (μV)	% Observed	100	100
	Mean; SD	1,010; 290.4	1,203; 367.1
	2→98 %	498→1,533	605→2,052

Modified from Rautaharju P, Rautaharju F. *Investigative electrocardiography in epidemiological studies and clinical trials*. London: Springer; 2007. p 1–289

[a]Includes for V1 and V2 R wave waves ≥25 V and for V3–V6 R waves ≥100 μV

Table A7 Limb lead amplitudes for larger S waves[a] in white and African-American women aged 40–59 years

Variable	Statistic	White (N=2,252)	African-American (N=778)
aVL S amplitude (μV)	% Observed	28	23
	Mean; SD	242; 130.4	228; 120.6
	2→98 %	102→634	102→606
I S amplitude (μV)	% Observed	23	15
	Mean; SD	177; 71.4	181; 68.5
	2→98 %	102→413	103→606
-aVR (inverted aVR)	% Observed	27	20
S amplitude (μV)	Mean; SD	160; 39.2	167; 64.8
	2→98 %	100→324	100→346
II S amplitude (μV)	% Observed	32	25
	Mean; SD	204; 102.4	228; 127.7
	2→98 %	102→516	102→673
aVF S amplitude (μV)	% Observed	31	31
	Mean; SD	226; 136.7	296; 195.6
	2→98 %	102→595	102→796
III S amplitude (μV)	% Observed	26	34
	Mean; SD	347; 264.5	514; 373.2
	2→98 %	102→1,108	107→1,403

Modified from Rautaharju P, Rautaharju F. *Investigative electrocardiography in epidemiological studies and clinical trials*. London: Springer; 2007. p 1–289

[a]Includes S waves ≥100 μV when R amplitude ≥100 μV

Table A8 ST J-point elevation amplitudes in limb leads for white and African-American women aged 40–59 years

Variable	Statistic	White (N=2,252)	African-American (N=778)
Lead I	% Observed	78	88
ST elevation (μV)	Mean; SD	20; 16.4	30;
	2→98 %	0→63	0→20
Lead II	% Observed	73	75
ST elevation (μV)	Mean; SD	27; 20.4	31; 23.5
	2→98 %	0→78	0→92
Lead III	% Observed	59	47
ST elevation (μV)	Mean; SD	23; 19.0	22; 19.9
	2→98 %	0→73	0→73
Lead aVR	% Observed	26	17
ST elevation (μV)	Mean; SD	10; 11.6	12; 13.9
	2→98 %	0→43	0→48
Lead aVL	% Observed	64	79
ST elevation (μV)	Mean; SD	19; 17.2	26; 20.9
	2→98 %	0→68	0→81
Lead aVF	% Observed	67	62
ST elevation (μV)	Mean; SD	24; 18.6	24; 20.5
	2→98 %	0→68	0→73

Modified from Rautaharju P, Rautaharju F. *Investigative electrocardiography in epidemiological studies and clinical trials*. London: Springer; 2007. p 1–289

Table A9 ST J-point depression amplitudes in limb leads for white and African-American women aged 40–59 years

Variable	Statistic	White (N=2,252)	African-American (N=778)
Lead I	% Observed	22	12
ST depression (μV)	Mean; SD	−16; 13.3	17; 16.5
	2→98 %	−59→−5	−54→−5
Lead II	% Observed	27	25
ST depression (μV)	Mean; SD	−22; 16.8	−24; 18.8
	2→98 %	−69→−5	−74→−5
Lead III	% Observed	41	53
ST depression (μV)	Mean; SD	−28; 21.5	−33; 25.2
	2→98 %	−88→−5	−93→−5
Lead aVR	% Observed	74	83
ST depression (μV)	Mean; SD	−24; 14.4	−30; 17.3
	2→98 %	−59→−5	−69→−5
Lead aVL	% Observed	36	21
ST depression (μV)	Mean; SD	−17; 12.5	−17; 13.4
	2→98 %	−49→−5	−50→−5
Lead aVF	% Observed	33	38
ST depression (μV)	Mean; SD	−24; 17.7	−27; 19.9
	2→98 %	−74→−5	−79→−5

Modified from Rautaharju P, Rautaharju F. *Investigative electrocardiography in epidemiological studies and clinical trials*. London: Springer; 2007. p 1–289

Table A10 ST J-point depression amplitudes in chest leads for white and African-American women aged 40–59 years

Variable	Statistic	White (N=2,252)	African-American (N=778)
LeadV1	% Observed	51	51
ST depression (μV)	Mean; SD	–21; 15.2	–25; 16.6
	2→98 %	–64→–5	–64→–5
Lead V2	% Observed	39	26
ST depression (μV)	Mean; SD	–27; 20.6	–25; 18.1
	2→98 %	–84→–5	–74→–5
Lead V3	% Observed	43	24
ST depression (μV)	Mean; SD	–28; 21.	–25; 21.6
	2→98 %	–84→–5	–85→–5
Lead V4	% Observed	46	25
ST depression (μV)	Mean; SD	–27; 21.5	–25; 24.4
	2→98 %	–86→–5	–83→–5
Lead V5	% Observed	40	22
ST depression (μV)	Mean; SD	–23; 19.0	–22; 23.0
	2→98 %	–79→–5	–69→–5
Lead V6	% Observed	26	17
ST depression (μV)	Mean; SD	–17; 15.5	–18; 18.1
	2→98 %	–59→–5	–50→–5

Modified from Rautaharju P, Rautaharju F. *Investigative electrocardiography in epidemiological studies and clinical trials*. London: Springer; 2007. p 1–289

Table A11 Amplitudes of uniphasic positive and negative[a] T waves in limb leads in white and African-American women aged 40–59 years

Variable	Statistic	White (N=2,252)	African-American (N=778)
Lead I	% Observed	96	95
Tpos. amplitude (μV)	Mean; SD	191; 84.1	185; 91.5
	2→98 %	35→385	0→400
Lead II	% Observed	97	96
Tpos. amplitude (μV)	Mean; SD	237; 92.2	198; 94.1
	2→98 %	68→449	0→419
Lead III	% Observed	67	52
Tpos. amplitude (μV)	Mean; SD	103; 71.0	89; 70.1
	2→98 %	0→273	0→263
Lead III	% Observed	33	48
Tneg. amplitude (μV)	Mean; SD	–67; 48.2	–76; 53.9
	2→98 %	–200→–14	–226→–14
Lead aVR	% Observed	97	94
Tneg. amplitude (μV)	Mean; SD	–215; 73.7	–194; 77.7
	2→98 %	–380→–83	–371→–63
Lead aVL	% Observed	83	87
Tpos. amplitude (μV)	Mean; SD	96; 65.9	106; 69.8
	2→98 %	0→258	0→283

(continued)

Table A.11 (continued)

Variable	Statistic	White (N=2,252)	African-American (N=778)
Lead aVL	% Observed	17	13
Tneg. amplitude (μV)	Mean; SD	−53; 42.6	−68; 60.2
	2→98 %	−170→−9	−240→−12
Lead aVF	% Observed	92	88
Tpos. amplitude (μV)	Mean; SD	155; 77.2	123; 74.7
	2→98 %	0→336	0→298
Lead aVF	% Observed	8	12
Tneg. amplitude (μV)	Mean; SD	−39; 27.9	−48; 33.4
	2→98 %	−119→−9	−145→−14

Modified from Rautaharju P, Rautaharju F. *Investigative electrocardiography in epidemiological studies and clinical trials*. London: Springer; 2007. p 1–289
[a]Includes T waves observed in over 5 %

Table A12 Uniphasic positive T wave amplitudes in chest leads including uniphasic negative and postive T in V1 and negative T-prime wave in V1 in white and African-American women aged 40–59 years

Variable	Statistic	White (N=2,252)	African-American (N=778)
LeadV1	% Observed	45	49
T neg. amplitude (μV)	Mean; SD	−95; 53.3	−95; 63.0
	2→98 %	−224→−14	−229→−14
LeadV1	% Observed	55	51
Tpos. amplitude (μV)	Mean; SD	97; 80.8	104; 89.6
	2→98 %	0→317	0→366
LeadV1	% Observed	6	4
T-prime neg. amplitude (μV)	Mean; SD	−57; 36.6	−50; 29.6
	2→98 %	−160→−9	−133→−9
Lead V2	% Observed	97	94
Tpos. amplitude (μV)	Mean; SD	327; 180.2	298; 167.2
	2→98 %	43→761	48→727
Lead V3	% Observed	98	96
Tpos. amplitude (μV)	Mean; SD	376; 189.7	318; 175.1
	2→98 %	68→814	58→761
Lead V4	% Observed	97	96
Tpos. amplitude (μV)	Mean; SD	349; 175.9	296; 163.7
	2→98 %	58→769	35→682
Lead V5	% Observed	97	95
Tpos. amplitude (μV)	Mean; SD	297; 145.9	258; 140.9
	2→98 %	43→649	24→605
Lead V6	% Observed	97	94
Tpos. amplitude (μV)	Mean; SD	227; 107.6	194; 107.9
	2→98 %	0→493	0→454

Modified from Rautaharju P, Rautaharju F. *Investigative electrocardiography in epidemiological studies and clinical trials*. London: Springer; 2007. p 1–289

Appendix B

Table B1 ST elevation amplitudes in limb leads in postmenopausal women by race

		White	Hispanic	African-American	Asian-Pacific Islander
I ST elevation (μV)	% Observed	81	86	93	83
	Mean; SD	21; 16.9	25; 18.8	34; 22.1	21; 16.3
	2→98 %	0→63	0→73	0→87	0→63
II ST elevation (μV)	% Observed	76	79	80	85
	Mean; SD	29; 20.8	30; 21.8	33; 23.4	32; 22.6
	2→98 %	0→78	0→78	0→87	0→87
III ST elevation (μV)	% Observed	58	53	47	66
	Mean; SD	23; 19.0	23; 19.5	21; 18.2	26; 19.7
	2→98 %	0→73	0→72	0→68	0→78
aVR ST elevation (μV)	% Observed	22	18	12	13
	Mean; SD	9; 9.8	7; 8.8	9; 12.1	7; 9.4
	2→98 %	0→34	0→34	0→42	0→33
aVL ST elevation (μV)	% Observed	66	72	82	81
	Mean; SD	19; 17.3	22; 18.5	28; 22.3	17; 15.9
	2→98 %	0→63	0→71	0→83	0→58
aVF ST elevation (μV)	% Observed	68	68	65	76
	Mean; SD	24; 19.0	25; 19.7	25; 19.5	28; 20.3
	2→98 %	0→73	0→68	0→73	0→81

Modified from Rautaharju et al. *J Electrocardiol.* 2013;46:707–16

P.M. Rautaharju, *The Female Electrocardiogram: Special Repolarization Features, Gender Differences, and the Risk of Adverse Cardiac Events*, DOI 10.1007/978-3-319-15293-6

Table B2 ST elevation amplitudes in chest leads in postmenopausal women by race

		White	Hispanic	African-American	Asian-Pacific Islander
		(N=31,060)	(N=1,700)	(N=2,721)	(N=818)
V1 ST elevation (μV)	% Observed	49	49	47	64
	Mean; SD	18; 18.2	18; 17.6	19; 21.0	20; 19.5
	2→98 %	0→69	0→68	0→73	0→68
V2 ST elevation (μV)	% Observed	63	70	80	80
	Mean; SD	35; 31.4	36; 30.2	45; 35.6	47; 36.7
	2→98 %	0→117	0→117	0→117	0→122
V3 ST elevation (μV)	% Observed	56	61	77	76
	Mean; SD	28; 25.5	29; 25.2	41; 32.0	39; 31.3
	2→98 %	0→97	0→92	0→83	0→102
V4 ST elevation (μV)	% Observed	56	63	78	72
	Mean; SD	25; 22.5	27; 23.4	38; 29.3	32; 27.1
	2→98 %	0→83	0→91	0→78	0→87
V5 ST elevation (μV)	% Observed	64	71	83	76
	Mean; SD	23; 19.6	25; 21.1	35; 25.2	26; 22.5
	2→98 %	0→73	0→78	0→68	0→78
V6 ST elevation (μV)	% Observed	79	82	89	83
	Mean; SD	22; 17.0	25; 18.2	31; 20.1	23; 18.1
	2→98 %	0→63	0→68	0→61.6	0→68

Modified from Rautaharju et al. *J Electrocardiol*. 2013;46:707–16

Table B3 ST depression amplitudes in limb leads in postmenopausal women by race

		White	Hispanic	African-American	Asian-Pacific Islander
I ST depression (μV)	% Observed	19	14	7	17
	Mean; SD	−13; 9.5	−12; 8.9	−14; 12.6	−12; 9.1
	2→98 %	−40→−5	−36→−5	−45→−5	−41→−5
II ST depression (μV)	% Observed	24	21	20	15
	Mean; SD	−21; 16.3	−21; 16.2	−22; 18.2	−17; 12.2
	2→98 %	−64→−5	−69→−5	−74→−5	−49→−5
III ST depression (μV)	% Observed	42	47	53	34
	Mean; SD	−28; 21.3	−29; 21.7	−35; 26.0	−24; 18.5
	2→98 %	−84→−5	−85→−5	−103→−5	−74→−5
aVR ST depression (μV)	% Observed	78	82	88	87
	Mean; SD	−25; 14.8	−28; 15.9	−33; 18.2	−27; 15.5
	2→98 %	−59→−5	−64→−5	−79→−5	−64→−5
aVL ST depression (μV)	% Observed	34	28	18	39
	Mean; SD	−16; 10.9	−16; 11.5	−15; 10.5	−16; 10.5
	2→98 %	−44→−5	−49→−5	−40→−5	−44→−5
aVF ST depression (μV)	% Observed	32	32	35	24
	Mean; SD	−23; 17.6	−23; 17.5	−27; 20.2	−19; 13.8
	2→98 %	−69→−5	−74→−5	−79→−5	−50→−5

Modified from Rautaharju et al. *J Electrocardiol*. 2013;46:707–16

Table B4 ST depression amplitudes in chest leads in postmenopausal women by race

		White	Hispanic	African-American	Asian-Pacific Islander
		(N=31,060)	(N=1,700)	(N=2,721)	(N=818)
V1 ST depression (μV)	% Observed	51	51	53	36
	Mean; SD	−21; 13.8	−22; 14.4	−22; 15.0	−19; 12.2
	2→98 %	−54→−5	−59→−5	−59→−5	−54→−5
V2 ST depression(μV)	% Observed	37	30	20	20
	Mean; SD	−26; 18.4	−24; 18.8	−22; 17.5	−21; 16.5
	2→98 %	−74→−5	−77→−6	−74→−5	−74→−5
V3 ST depression (μV)	% Observed	44	39	23	24
	Mean; SD	−26; 17.8	−24; 17.0	−23; 18.7	−22; 15.6
	2→98 %	−74→−5	−69→−5	−91→−5	−69→−5
V4 ST depression (μV)	% Observed	44	37	22	28
	Mean; SD	−24; 16.6	−23; 15.4	−22; 19.5	−20; 14.6
	2→98 %	−64→−5	−64→−5	−74→−5	−64→−5
V5 ST depression (μV)	% Observed	36	29	17	24
	Mean; SD	−20; 13.9	−19; 12.9	−19; 17.3	−18; 14.0
	2→98 %	−54→−5	−54→−5	−74→−5	−54→−5
V6 ST depression (μV)	% Observed	21	18	11	17
	Mean; SD	15; 10.7	−15; 11.7	−15; 14.1	−13; 10.6
	2→98 %	−44→−5	−48→−5	−54→−5	−44→−5

Modified from Rautaharju et al. *J Electrocardiol.* 2013;46:707–16

Table B5 Amplitudes of uniphasic positive T waves in limb leads and uniphasic negative T waves in leads III and aVR in postmenopausal women by race

		White	Hispanic	African-American	Asian-Pacific Islander
Lead I Tpos.	% Observed	99	99	98	100
Amplitude(μV)	Mean; SD	215; 88.4	225; 92.2	215;100.5	217; 89.8
	2→98 %	58→419	57→439	53→419	53→410
Lead II Tpos.	% Observed	99	99	98	100
Amplitude(μV)	Mean; SD	264; 95.6	250; 95.2	228; 101.9	262; 104.5
	2→98 %	87→478	78→459	78→458	58→483
Lead III Tpos	% Observed	68	61	54	64
Amplitude(μV)	Mean; SD	105; 72.0	93; 66.2	89; 67.4	107; 73.9
	2→98 %	0→283	0→236	0→288	0→296
Lead aVL	% Observed	87	90	92	92
T amplitude(μV)	Mean; SD	104; 69.4	118; 73.3	118; 76.4	105; 67.9
	2→98 %	0→278	0→302	0→278	0→263
Lead aVF	% Observed	96	95	91	96
T amplitude(μV)	Mean; SD	167; 80.7	150; 78.5	138; 77.7	165; 85.9
	2→98 %	0→356	0→332	0→351	0→358
Lead III Tneg	% Observed	32	39	46	36
	Mean; SD	−69; 49.9	−69; 49.9	−83; 56.0	−68; 47.4
	2→98 %	−205→−14	−228→−14	−205→−14	−190→−14
Lead aVR Tneg.	% Observed	99	99	97	98
Amplitude(μV)	Mean; SD	−241; 76.8	−241; 76.8	−225; 85.5	−243; 81.2
	2→98 %	−410→−97	−415→−90	−395→−103	−424→−97

Modified from Rautaharju et al. *J Electrocardiol.* 2013;46:707–16

Table B6 ST J-point elevation amplitudes in chest leads for white and African-American women aged 40–59 years

Variable	Statistic	White (N=2,252)	African-American (N=778)
LeadV1	% Observed	49	49
ST elevation (μV)	Mean; SD	20; 20.7	21; 20.1
	2→98 %	0→78	0→73
Lead V2	% Observed	61	74
ST elevation (μV)	Mean; SD	34; 31.2	43; 35.5
	2→98 %	0→117	0→141
Lead V3	% Observed	57	76
ST elevation (μV)	Mean; SD	28; 25.7	40; 30.5
	2→98 %	0→97	0→120
Lead V4	% Observed	54	75
ST elevation (μV)	Mean; SD	24; 22.6	37; 27.1
	2→98 %	0→83	0→106
Lead V5	% Observed	60	78
ST elevation (μV)	Mean; SD	22; 20.0	33; 24.5
	2→98 %	0→73	0→92
Lead V6	% Observed	74	83
ST elevation (μV)	Mean; SD	22; 17.1	29; 20.3
	2→98 %	0→63	0→83

Modified from Rautaharju P, Rautaharju F. *Investigative electrocardiography in epidemiological studies and clinical trials*. London: Springer; 2007. p 1–289

Table B7 Amplitudes of uniphasic positive T waves in chest leads including V1 lead uniphasic negative T waves and V1 Tprime waves in postmenopausal women

		White	Hispanic	African-American	Asian-Pacific Islander
Lead V1 Tneg.	% Observed	55	52	54	63
Amplitude(μV)	Mean; SD	−101; 55.4	−95; 53.7	−103; 58.0	−103; 56.0
	2→98 %	−239→−19	−231→−19	−244→−19	−243→−19
Lead V1 Tpos.	% Observed	38	39	40	33
Amplitude(μV)	Mean; SD	88; 73.7	94; 69.3	100; 85.9	88; 71.6
	2→98 %	0→283	0→266	0→332	0→271
Lead V1 Tprime.	% Observed	6	9	5	0
Amplitude(μV)	Mean; SD	−51; 29.0	−46; 27.9	−49; 28.6	
	2→98 %	−126→−9	−123→−9	−129→−8	
Lead V2 Tpos.	% Observed	97	98	97	97
Amplitude(μV)	Mean; SD	137; 177.8	329; 170.0	321; 168.3	326; 174.9
	2→98 %	43→756	58→732	18→766	63→748
Lead V3 Tpos	% Observed	99	98	97	98
Amplitude(μV)	Mean; SD	383; 185.9	350; 183.6	329; 178.8	389; 195.6
	2→98 %	63→810	53→798	35→800	83→874
Lead V4 Tpos	% Observed	99	99	98	99
Amplitude(μV)	Mean; SD	364; 174.8	337; 173.8	315; 174.0	382; 191.9
	2→98 %	63→776	42→747	29→781	73→859
Lead V5 Tpos	% Observed	99	99	98	99
Amplitude(μV)	Mean; SD	316; 164.4	301; 148.8	277; 154.1	344; 166.7
	2→98 %	63→659	46→634	43→673	68→740
Lead V6 Tpos	% Observed	99	99	97	99
Amplitude(μV)	Mean; SD	242; 107.0	241; 114.1	212; 117.3	273;124.9
	2→98 %	53→498	0→504	15→502	48→546

Modified from Rautaharju et al. *J Electrocardiol*. 2013;46:707–16

Appendix C

Table C1 Gender differences in normal ranges for heart rate, PR interval, QRS duration and rate-adjusted QT interval by race and age

Variable	White			
	Age 40–49 years		Age 60 years and older	
	Women (N=2,252)	Men (N=1,478)	Women (N=3,312)	Men (N=2,337)
Heart rate/min	51→90	48→91	49→92	46→92
PR interval (ms)	124→202	126→210	120→218	128→226
QRS interval (ms)	72→104	78→114	68→104	74→114
TpTe interval[a] (ms)	60→118	70→132	60→128	66→142
QTea[b] (ms)	388→448	382→436	391→456	385→449
	African-American			
	Age 40–49 years		Age 60 years and older	
	Women (N=452)	Men (N=778)	Women (N=459)	Men (N=639)
Heart rate/min	50→92	49→93	48→94	48→95
PR interval (ms)	124→216	124→220	122→226	126→226
QRS interval (ms)	70→104	76→112	68→108	72→112
TpTe interval[a] (ms)	58→132	70→144	46→150	60→146
QTea[b] (ms)	385→449	378→442	388→458	381→454

[a]TpTe is the interval from global T wave peak (Tp) to Tend (Te)

[b]QTea is the QTend interval rate-adjusted as a linear function of RR interval whereby QTea = QTe −168*(RR-1) for women and QTea = QTe − 154*(RR-1) for men

P.M. Rautaharju, *The Female Electrocardiogram: Special Repolarization Features, Gender Differences, and the Risk of Adverse Cardiac Events*,
DOI 10.1007/978-3-319-15293-6

Table C2 Gender differences in normal ranges for P wave durations and amplitudes by race, age and gender

Variable	White			
	Age 40–49 years		Age 60 years and older	
	Women	Men	Women	Men
	(N=2,252)	(N=1,478)	(N=3,312)	(N=2,337)
PII duration (ms)				
Present (%)	100	99	99	98
Range[a]	80→126	86→132	66→134	73→140
PII amplitude (μV)				
Present (%)	100	99	98	97
Range	43→205	43→15	39→200	34→185
PV1 duration (ms)	28→118	32→120	27→118	30→118
Present (%)	99	100	99	97
Range	28→118	32→120	27→118	30→118
PV1 amplitude (μV)				
Present (%)	95	98	91	93
Range	14→87	14→97	9→102	9→102
P′V1[b] duration (ms)				
Present (%)	55	61	75	75
Range	29→82	30→83	33→88	36→91
P′V1[b] amplitude (μV)				
Present (%)	60	59	81	80
Range	−83→−19	−96→−24	−98→−24	−97→−24
	African-American			
	Age 40–49 years		Age 60 years and older	
	Women	Men	Women	Men
	(N=452)	(N=778)	(N=459)	(N=639)
PII duration (ms)				
Present (%)	100	100	99	98
Range	86→132	90→138	85→138	86→144
PII amplitude (μV)				
Present (%)	99	100	98	97
Range	43→209	43→219	41→222	39→239
PV1 duration (ms)				
Present (%)	99	99	99	98
Range	30→124	30→124	28→118	28→122
PV1 amplitude (μV)				
Present (%)	98	98	95	93
Range	14→101	18→119	14→102	14→104
P′V1[b] duration (ms)				
Present (%)	60	59	81	81
Range	39→87	24→93	67→125	40→96
P′V1[b] amplitude (μV)				
Present (%)	60	59	81	808
Range	−97→−24	−110→−24	−117→−24	−105→−24

[a]Range is from 2nd to 98th percentile of the distribution
[b]P′V1 is the P prime wave; P′V1 amplitude and duration listed only for biphasic positive/negative P waves

Table C3 Gender differences in normal ranges for Q wave durations and amplitudes[a] by race and age

	White			
	Age 40–49 years		Age 60 years and older	
	Women	Men	Women	Men
Lead/variable	(N=2,252)	(N=1,478)	(N=3,312)	(N=2,337)
aVL Q duration (ms)				
Present (%)	31	44	45	48
Range	13→29	14→30	11→30	13→32
I Q duration (ms)				
Present (%)	44	52	47	47
Range	12→26	13→27	12→27	13→28
II Q duration (ms)				
Present (%)	49	41	32	30
Range	11→26	12→28	11→27	12→29
aVF Q duration (ms)				
Present (%)	46	37	28	26
Range	12→31	12→34	11→38	12→41
III Q duration (ms)				
Present (%)	44	33	26	25
Range	12→44	13→49	12→51	13→54
V4 Q duration (ms)				
Present (%)	20	23	25	21
Range	11→24	11→25	10→24	10→25
V5 Q duration (ms)				
Present (%)	41	50	41	39
Range	11→25	12→27	10→25	11→26
V6 Q duration (ms)				
Present (%)	60	59	51	46
Range	12→26	13→28	11→25	12→27
	African-American			
	Age 40–49 years		Age 60 years and older	
	Women	Men	Women	Men
Lead/variable	(N=452)	(N=778)	(N=459)	(N=639)
aVL Q duration (ms)				
Present (%)	46	50	57	52
Range	12→27	13→27	12→35	11→31
I Q duration (ms)				
Present (%)	45	46	47	42
Range	11→24	13→25	11→37	12→26
II Q duration (ms)				
Present (%)	23	25	20	21
Range	10→27	12→28	10→31	12→30
aVF Q duration (ms)				
Present (%)	25	24	20	18

(continued)

Table C3 (continued)

	African-American			
	Age 40–49 years		Age 60 years and older	
	Women	Men	Women	Men
Lead/variable	(N=452)	(N=778)	(N=459)	(N=639)
Range	11→30	11→32	11→37	12→31
III Q duration (ms)				
Present (%)	27	22	18	19
Range	12→45	11→47	11→50	13→53
V4 Q duration (ms)				
Present (%)	16	23	20	23
Range	10→22	10→23	10→25	9→23
V5 Q duration (ms)				
Present (%)	32	42	34	35
Range	11→24	11→25	11→36	11→24
V6 Q duration (ms)				
Present (%)	45	48	40	37
Range	12→25	13→27	11→41	12→25

[a]Includes Q waves with amplitude ≥25 μV combined with R amplitude ≥100 μV

Table C4 Gender differences in normal ranges for R wave amplitudes[a] in limb leads by race and age

	White			
	Age 40–49 years		Age 60 years and older	
	Women	Men	Women	Men
Lead	(N=2,252)	(N=1,478)	(N=3,312)	(N=2,337)
aVL				
Present (%)	82	89	93	93
Range[b]	112→1,065	119→1,235	122→1,299	126→1,259
I				
Present (%)	100	100	100	100
Range	129→1,411	263→1,511	268→1,512	224→1,464
II				
Present (%)	100	99	99	97
Range	332→1,629	239→1,629	190→1,435	146→1,360
aVF				
Present (%)	94	86	83	76
Range	131→1,331	112→1,396	112→1,149	107→1,134

(continued)

Table C4 (continued)

Lead	White			
	Age 40–49 years		Age 60 years and older	
	Women	Men	Women	Men
	(N=2,252)	(N=1,478)	(N=3,312)	(N=2,337)
III				
Present (%)	74	66	58	57
Range	107→1,186	102→1,259	102→1,051	102→976

Lead	African-American			
	Age 40–49 years		Age 60 years and older	
	Women	Men	Women	Men
	(N=452)	(N=778)	(N=459)	(N=639)
aVL				
Present (%)	92	92	97	93
Range[b]	123→1,313	131→1,454	179→1,598	126→1,371
I				
Present (%)	100	100	100	100
Range	339→1,625	361→1,655	425→1,821	274→1,625
II				
Present (%)	99	98	99	97
Range	291→1,832	287→1,907	198→1,716	178→1,667
aVF				
Present (%)	93	87	85	94
Range	126→1,431	130→1,655	112→1,289	112→1,296
III				
Present (%)	71	69	63	63
Range	102→1,156	107→1,428	102→1,110	107→1,140

[a]Includes R waves ≥100 μV

[b]Range from 2nd to 98th percentile of the distribution

Table C5 Gender differences in normal ranges for R wave amplitudes[a] in chest leads by race and age

	White			
	Age 40–49 years		Age 60 years and older	
	Women	Men	Women	Men
Lead	(N=2,252)	(N=1,478)	(N=3,312)	(N=2,337)
V1				
Present (%)	96	97	90	89
Range[b]	39→502	43→566	34→527	34→522
V2				
Present (%)	100	100	98	99
Range	87→1,147	107→1,497	63→1,425	63→1,536
V3				
Present (%)	99	100	99	99
Range	175→1,743	239→2,172	127→2,230	185→2,303
V4				
Present (%)	100	100	100	100
Range	415→2,172	605→2,763	451→2,651	453→2,880
V5				
Present (%)	100	100	100	100
Range[b]	532→2,041	678→2,638	528→2,641	576→2,695
V6				
Present (%)	100	100	100	100
Range	498→1,704	468→1,845	429→2,049	374→1,967
	African-American			
	Age 40–49 years		Age 60 years and older	
	Women	Men	Women	Men
Lead	(N=152)	(N=778)	(N=459)	(N=639)
V1				
Present (%)	96	94	87	86
Range[b]	34→522	34→853	34→632	34→869
V2				
Present (%)	99	100	98	98
Range	87→1,206	92→1,762	58→1,808	58→1,718
V3				
Present (%)	99	100	99	98
Range	200→1,937	288→2,928	219→2,597	219→2,824
V4				
Present (%)	100	100	100	100
Range	466	2,519	748	3,393
V5				
Present (%)	100	100	100	100
Range	377→2,570	771→2,846	660→2,829	739→3,419
V6				
Present (%)	100	100	100	100
Range	605→2,052	537→2,001	510→2,309	463→2,200

[a]Includes R waves ≥25 μV for V1 and V2 and R waves ≥100 μV for V3–V6
[b]Range from 2nd to 98th percentile of the distribution

Table C6 Gender differences in normal ranges for S wave amplitudes[a] in limb leads by race and age

Lead	White			
	Age 40–49 years		Age 60 years and older	
	Women (N=2,252)	Men (N=1,478)	Women (N=3,312)	Men (N=2,337)
aVL				
Present (%)	28	69	19	25
Range[b]	102→634	102→651	102→582	102→499
I				
Present (%)	23	39	15	23
Range	102→413	102→439	102→375	102→341
II				
Present (%)	32	38	36	40
Range	102→516	102→566	102→620	102→670
aVF				
Present (%)	31	29	35	32
Range	102→595	105→685	102→937	102→912
III				
Present (%)	23	27	30	28
Range	102→1,108	107→1,314	107→1,496	107→1,445
	African-American			
	Age 40–49 years		Age 60 years and older	
Lead	Women (N=452)	Men (N=778)	Women (N=459)	Men (N=639)
aVL				
Present (%)	23	34	18	24
Range[b]	102→606	102→649	102→568	107→575
I				
Present (%)	15	28	11	16
Range	103→373	104→429	102→382	102→352
II				
Present (%)	25	34	35	40
Range	102→573	107→678	105→771	105→711
aVF				
Present (%)	31	34	41	41
Range	102→796	107→922	108→1,214	107→1,018
III				
Present (%)	34	35	40	50
Range	107→1,403	108→1,504	122→2,000	105→1,509

[a]Includes S waves ≥100 μV if R wave amplitude ≥100 μV
[b]Range from 2nd to 98th percentile of the distribution

Table C7 Gender differences in normal ranges for S wave amplitudes[a] in chest leads by race and age

	White			
	Age 40–49 years		Age 60 years and older	
	Women	Men	Women	Men
Lead	(N=2,252)	(N=1,478)	(N=3,312)	(N=2,337)
V1				
Present (%)	75	80	60	60
Range[b]	292→1,616	242→1,699	272→1,624	213→1,658
V2				
Present (%)	96	98	93	94
Range	317→1,990	361→2,291	255→2,011	288→2,223
V3				
Present (%)	97	98	96	97,161
Range	161→1,401	200→1,847	161→1,584	211→1,912
V4				
Present (%)	89	91	87	93
Range	117→937	117→1,309	117→1,135	131→1,502
V5				
Present (%)	65	62	58	68
Range[b]	102→629	109→752	102→756	107→889
V6				
Present (%)	21	27	20	29
Range	102→428	107→459	102→512	102→504
	African-American			
	Age 40–49 years		Age 60 years and older	
	Women	Men	Women	Men
Lead	(N=452)	(N=778)	(N=459)	(N=639)
V1				
Present (%)	75	76	55	59
Range[b]	398→2,015	317→2,384	361→2,028	293→2,524
V2				
Present (%)	96	96	94	92
Range	379→2,232	348→2,707	253→2,373	296→2,598
V3				
Present (%)	94	94	94	93
Range	141→1,426	200→2,131	146→1,770	200→2,307
V4				
Present (%)	82	83	83	87
Range	117→1,026	126→1,403	112→1,255	141→1,791
V5				
Present (%)	59	55	57	58
Range	107→702	107→876	107→958	109→812
V6				
Present (%)	20	22	18	23
Range	102→510	102→513	107→682	102→443

[a]Includes S waves ≥100 μV if R wave amplitude ≥100 μV

[b]Range from 2nd to 98th percentile of the distribution

Table C8 Gender differences in normal ranges for ST J-point elevation in limb leads by race and age

	White			
	Age 40–59 years		Age 60 years and older	
	Women	Men	Women	Men
Lead/variable	(N=2,252)	(N=1,478)	(N=3,312)	(N=2,337)
aVL ST elevation (μV)				
Present (%)	61	62	59	62
Range[a]	0→69	0→66	0→73	0→73
I ST elevation (μV)				
Present (%)	85	80	78	82
Range	0→71	0→70	0→68	0→73
aVR ST depression[b] (μV)				
Present (%)	88	83	81	83
Range	−69→0	−64→0	−64→0	−69→0
II ST elevation (μV)				
Present (%)	79	73	72	74
Range	0→88	0→83	0→83	0→86
aVF ST elevation (μV)				
Present (%)	71	64	64	65
Range	0→78	0→73	0→73	0→78
III ST elevation (μV)				
Present (%)	59	56	55	55
Range	0→73	0→76	0→73	0→73
	African-American			
	Women		Men	
	(N=452)		(N=778)	
	Women	Men	Women	Men
	(N=452)	(N=778)	(N=459)	(N=639)
aVL ST elevation (μV)				
Present (%)	62	62	64	55
Range	0→73	0→72	0→71	0→66
I ST elevation (μV)				
Present (%)	62	79	82	74
Range	0→68	0→73	0→71	0→68
aVR ST depression (μV)				
Present (%)	83	80	83	79
Range	−64→0	−69→0	−64→0	−63→0
II ST elevation (μV)				
Present (%)	73	69	73	72
Range	0→78	0→83	0→83	0→80
aVF ST elevation (μV)				
Present (%)	64	61	62	67
Range	0→68	0→73	0→73	0→72
III ST elevation (μV)				
Present (%)	56	53	50	57
Range	0→70	0→73	0→81	0→72

[a]Range is from 2nd to 98th percentile of the distribution
[b]ST depression in aVR corresponds to ST elevation in left lateral leads

Table C9 Gender differences in normal ranges for ST J-point elevation in chest leads by race and age

	White			
	Age 40–59 years		Age 60 years and older	
	Women	Men	Women	Men
Lead/variable	(N=2,252)	(N=1,478)	(N=3,312)	(N=2,337)
V1 ST elevation (μV)				
Present (%)	54	55	57	57
Range[a]	0→92	0→83	0→92	0→87
V2 ST elevation (μV)				
Present (%)	72	71	71	74
Range	0→151	0→136	0→151	0→166
V3 ST elevation (μV)				
Present (%)	72	67	66	71
Range	0→141	0→122	0→141	0→150
V4 ST elevation (μV)				
Present (%)	71	57	59	66
Range	0→122	0→102	0→112	0→126
V5 ST elevation (μV)				
Present (%)	75	64	63	68
Range	0→97	0→37	0→87	0→92
V6 elevation (μV)				
Present (%)	82	77	74	76
Range	0→78	0→68	0→73	0→73
	African-American			
	Age 40–59 years		Age 60 years and older	
	Women	Men	Women	Men
	(N=452)	(N=778)	(N=459)	(N=639)
V1 ST elevation (μV)				
Present (%)	52	57	56	55
Range	0→87	0→83	0→83	0→78
V2 ST elevation (μV)				
Present (%)	67	73	73	63
Range	0→129	0→138	0→161	0→142
V3 ST elevation (μV)				
Present (%)	68	66	66	58
Range	0→122	0→126	0→159	0→1,360
V4 ST elevation (μV)				
Present (%)	60	61	60	54
Range	0→107	0→95	0→128	0→103
V5 ST elevation (μV)				
Present (%)	65	82	64	56
Range	0→87	0→80	0→92	0→87
V6 ST elevation (μV)				
Present (%)	78	75	73	67
Range	0→73	0→78	0→76	0→68

[a]Range is from 2nd to 98th percentile of the distribution
[b]ST depression in aVR corresponds to ST elevation in left lateral leads

Table C10 Gender differences in normal ranges for ST J-point depression in limb leads by race and age

Lead/variable	White			
	Age 40–59 years		Age 60 years and older	
	Women	Men	Women	Men
	(N=2,252)	(N=1,478)	(N=3,312)	(N=2,337)
aVL ST depression(μV)				
Present (%)	39	38	41	38
Range[a]	−44→−5	−49→−5	−52→−5	−49→−5
I ST depression (μV)				
Present (%)	15	20	22	18
Range	−40→−5	−54→−5	−59→−5	−59→−5
aVR ST elevation[b] (μV)				
Present (%)	82	76	74	77
Range	0→69	−64→−5	0→64	−69→−5
II ST depression (μV)				
Present (%)	21	27	28	26
Range	−69→−5	−69→−5	−74→−5	−74→−5
aVF ST depression (μV)				
Present (%)	29	36	36	35
Range	−74→−5	−69→−5	−79→−5	−79→−5
III ST depression (μV)				
Present (%)	41	44	45	45
Range	−85→−5	−84→−5	−88→−5	−98→−5
	African-American			
	Age 40–59 years		Age 60 years and older	
	Women	Men	Women	Men
	(N=452)	(N=778)	(N=459)	(N=639)
aVL ST depression(μV)				
Present (%)	38	38	36	45
Range[a]	−50→−5	−50→−5	−5→−54	−50→−5
I ST depression (μV)				
Present (%)	18	21	18	26
Range	−55→−5	−56→−5	−56→−5	−50→−5
aVR ST elevation[b] (μV)				
Present (%)	76	75	76	71
Range	0→64	0→69	0→65	−64→−5
II ST depression (μV)				
Present (%)	27	31	27	28
Range	−78→−5	−80→−5	−74→−5	−56→−5
aVF ST depression (μV)				
Present (%)	36	39	38	33
Range	−78→−5	−78→−5	−64→−5	−70→−5
III ST elevation (μV)				
Present (%)	44	47	50	43
Range	−99→−5	−97→−5	−84→−5	−84→−5

[a]Range is from 2nd to 98th percentile of the distribution
[b]ST elevation in aVR corresponds to ST depression in left lateral leads

Table C11 Gender differences in normal ranges for ST J-point elevation in chest leads by race and age

Lead/variable	White			
	Age 40–59 years		Age 60 years and older	
	Women	Men	Women	Men
	(N=2,252)	(N=1,478)	(N=3,312)	(N=2,337)
V1 ST depression (μV)				
Present (%)	46	45	43	43
Range[a]	−64→−5	−63→−5	−64→5	−59→−5
V2 ST depression (μV)				
Present (%)	28	29	29	
Range	−64→−5	−91→−5	−84→−5	−83→−5
V3 ST depression (μV)				
Present (%)	28	33	34	
Range	−64→−5	−101→−5	−93→−5	−79→−5
V4 ST depression (μV)				
Present (%)	28	43	41	
Range	−54→−5	−93→−5	−93→−5	−84→−5
V5 ST depression (μV)				
Present (%)	25	36	37	
Range	−49→−5	−81→−5	−79→−5	−70→−5
V6 depression (μV)				
Present (%)	18	23	26	
Range	−35→−5	−69→−5	−64→−5	−54→−5
	African-American			
	Age 40–59 years		Age 60 years and older	
	Women	Men	Women	Men
	(N=452)	(N=778)	(N=459)	(N=639)
V1 ST depression (μV)				
Present (%)	46	45	44	45
Range	−64→−5	−63→−5	−64→−5	−58→−5
V2 ST depression (μV)				
Present (%)	28	29	27	37
Range	−64→−5	−91→−5	−84→−5	−64→−5
V3 ST depression (μV)				
Present (%)	28	33	34	42
Range	−64→−5	−89→−5	−88→−5	−70→−5
V4 ST depression (μV)				
Present (%)	29	43	40	46
Range	−54→−5	−93→−5	−93→−5	−79→−5
V5 ST depression (μV)				
Present (%)	25	36	36	44
Range	−49→−5	−81→−5	−68→−5	−93→−5
V6 ST depression (μV)				
Present (%)	18	23	27	33
Range	−35→−5	−69→−5	−60→−5	−64→−5

[a]Range is from 2nd to 98th percentile of the distribution

Table C12 Gender differences in normal ranges for uniphasic T waves in limb leads by race and age

Lead/variable	White			
	Age 40–59 years		Age 60 years and older	
	Women (N=2,252)	Men (N=1,478)	Women (N=3,312)	Men (N=2,337)
aVL Tpos. (μV)				
Present (%)	90	82	81	85
Range[a]	0→288	0→278	0→278	0→268
I ST Tpos. (μV)				
Present (%)	99	96	96	96
Range	0→417	29→422	0→395	0→385
aVR Tneg.[b] (μV)				
Present (%)	98	96	96	96
Range	−385→−73	−385→−73	−385→−73	−371→−68
II Tpos. (μV)				
Present (%)	99	97	97	97
Range	68→468	48→454	21→447	4→444
aVF Tpos. (μV)				
Present (%)	93	93	92	90
Range	0→346	0→346	0→341	0→332
III Tpos. (μV)				
Present (%)	61	65	65	60
Range	0→292	0→283	0→292	0→273
	African-American			
	Age 40–59 years		Age 60 years and older	
	Women (N=452)	Men (N=778)	Women (N=459)	Men (N=639)
aVL Tpos. (μV)				
Present (%)	82	79	85	85
Range[a]	0→279	0→263	0→273	0→280
I ST Tpos. (μV)				
Present (%)	95	95	95	97
Range	33→386	39→405	0→405	20→397
aVR Tneg.[b] (μV)				
Present (%)	96	95	95	97
Range	−380→−78	−410→−71	−385→−78	−386→−68
II Tpos. (μV)				
Present (%)	97	95	96	98
Range	44→444	0→506	0→437	48→483
aVF Tpos. (μV)				
Present (%)	90	90	89	93
Range	0→346	0→379	0→322	0→358
III Tpos. (μV)				
Present (%)	63	62	60	63
Range	0→289	0→336	0→263	0→291

[a]Range is from 2nd to 98th percentile of the distribution
[b]Uniphasic Tneg. in aVR corresponds to uniphasic Tpos in left lateral leads

Table C13 Gender differences in normal ranges for T waves in chest leads by race and age

Lead/variable	White			
	Age 40–59 years		Age 60 years and older	
	Women (N=2,252)	Men (N=1,478)	Women (N=3,312)	Men (N=2,337)
V1 uniphasic Tneg. (μV)				
Present (%)	40	32	31	34
Range[a]	−224→−14	−226→−19	−224→−14	−214→−14
V1 uniphasic Tos. (μV)				
Present (%)	55	60	63	62
Range	0→385	0→420	0→456	0→463
V1 T′neg.[b] (μV)				
Present (%)	5	7	6	4
Range	−122→−9	−170→−9	−163→−9	−109→−9
V2 Tpos. (μV)				
Present (%)	98	97	98	98
Range	48→913	58→987	68→961	73→954
V3 Tpos. (μV)				
Present (%)	99	98	98	99
Range	73→959	78→1,025	92→996	63→844
V4 Tpos. (μV)				
Present (%)	99	98	97	98
Range	78→864	67→899	68→868	63→844
V5 Tpos. (μV)				
Present (%)	99	96	96	96
Range	68→668	53→691	24→673	34→644
V6 Tpos. (μV)				
Present (%)	99	96	96	96
Range	53→498	0→499	0→498	0→454
	African-American			
	Age 40–59 years		Age 60 years and older	
	Women (N=452)	Men (N=778)	Women (N=459)	Men (N=639)
V1 uniphasic Tneg. (μV)				
Present (%)	30	29	32	40
Range[a]	−221→−14	−238→−14	−239→−14	−224→−24
V1 uniphasic Tos. (μV)				
Present (%)	63	64	64	56
Range	0→440	0→363	0→375	0→463
V1 T′neg.[b] (μV)				
Present (%)	7	6	4	4
Range	−122→−9	−148→−14	−106→−21	−136→−16
V2 Tpos. (μV)				
Present (%)	97	98	97	96
Range	83→936	67→866	25→901	62→864

(continued)

Table C13 (continued)

	African-American			
	Age 40–59 years		Age 60 years and older	
	Women	Men	Women	Men
	(N=452)	(N=778)	(N=459)	(N=639)
V3 Tpos. (μV)				
Present (%)	98	98	97	97
Range	108→960	80→927	6→955	72→867
V4 Tpos. (μV)				
Present (%)	97	97	96	97
Range	64→863	53→831	5→855	53→839
V5 Tpos. (μV)				
Present (%)	96	96	95	97
Range	52→659	24→673	0→687	23→650
V6 Tpos. (μV)				
Present (%)	96	96	95	96
Range	38→489	0→498	0→498	0→473

[a]Range is from 2nd to 98th percentile of the distribution
[b]V1 T′neg. is the negative Tprime amplitude of a pos./neg. T wave

Index

P.M. Rautaharju, *The Female Electrocardiogram: Special Repolarization Features, Gender Differences, and the Risk of Adverse Cardiac Events*,
DOI 10.1007/978-3-319-15293-6

MIX
Papier aus verantwortungsvollen Quellen
Paper from responsible sources
FSC® C105338

If you have any concerns about our products,
you can contact us on
ProductSafety@springernature.com

In case Publisher is established outside the EU,
the EU authorized representative is:
Springer Nature Customer Service Center GmbH
Europaplatz 3, 69115 Heidelberg, Germany

Printed by Libri Plureos GmbH
in Hamburg, Germany